Advances in Equine Imaging

Editors

NATASHA M. WERPY
MYRA F. BARRETT

VETERINARY CLINICS OF NORTH AMERICA: EQUINE PRACTICE

www.vetequine.theclinics.com

Consulting Editor
ANTHONY SIMON TURNER

December 2012 • Volume 28 • Number 3

ELSEVIER

1600 John F. Kennedy Boulevard • Suite 1800 • Philadelphia, Pennsylvania 19103

http://www.vetequine.theclinics.com

VETERINARY CLINICS OF NORTH AMERICA: EQUINE PRACTICE Volume 28, Number 3
December 2012 ISSN 0749-0739, ISBN-13: 978-1-4557-4967-6

Editor: John Vassallo; j.vassallo@elsevier.com
Developmental Editor: Teia Stone

Veterinary Clinics of North America: Equine Practice (ISSN 0749-0739) is published in April, August, and December by Elsevier Inc., 360 Park Avenue South, New York, NY 10010-1710. Business and Editorial Offices: 1600 John F. Kennedy Blvd., Suite 1800, Philadelphia, PA 19103-2899. Subscription prices are $267.00 per year (domestic individuals), $397.00 per year (domestic institutions), $126.00 per year (domestic students/residents), $299.00 per year (Canadian individuals), $496.00 per year (Canadian institutions), $346.00 per year (international individuals), $496.00 per year (international institutions), and $172.00 per year (international and Canadian students/residents). To receive student/resident rate, orders must be accompanied by name of affiliated institution, date of term, and the signature of program/residency coordinator on institution letterhead. Orders will be billed at individual rate until proof of status is received. Foreign air speed delivery is included in all *Clinics* subscription prices. All prices are subject to change without notice. **POSTMASTER:** Send address changes to *Veterinary Clinics of North America: Equine Practice*, 3251 Riverport Lane, Maryland Heights, MO 63043. Customer Service (orders, claims, online, change of address): Elsevier Health Sciences Division, Subscription Customer Service, 3251 Riverport Lane, Maryland Heights, MO 63043. Tel: 1-800-654-2452 (U.S. and Canada); 314-447-8871 (outside U.S. and Canada). Fax: 314-447-8029. E-mail: journalscustomer service-usa@elsevier.com (for print support); E-mail: journalsonlinesupport-usa@elsevier (for online support).

Reprints. For copies of 100 or more of articles in this publication, please contact the Commercial Reprints Department, Elsevier Inc., 360 Park Avenue South, New York, NY 10010-1710. Tel.: 212-633-3812; Fax: 212-462-1935; E-mail: reprints@elsevier.com.

Veterinary Clinics of North America: Equine Practice is covered in *MEDLINE/PubMed (Index Medicus), Excerpta Medica, Current Contents/Agriculture, Biology and Environmental Sciences, and ISI.*

Printed and bound by CPI Group (UK) Ltd, Croydon, CR0 4YY

Transferred to digital print 2012

Contributors

CONSULTING EDITOR

ANTHONY SIMON TURNER, BVSc, MS
Diplomate, American College of Veterinary Surgeons; Professor, Department of Clinical Sciences, College of Veterinary Medicine and Biomedical Sciences, Colorado State University, Fort Collins, Colorado

GUEST EDITORS

NATASHA M. WERPY, DVM
Diplomate, American College of Veterinary Radiology; Associate Professor, Diagnostic Imaging; Small Animal Clinical Sciences, Radiology Department, College of Veterinary Medicine, University of Florida, Gainesville, Florida

MYRA F. BARRETT, DVM, MS
Diplomate, American College of Veterinary Radiology; Assistant Professor of Radiology, Department of Environmental and Radiological Health Sciences, Veterinary Teaching Hospital, Colorado State University, Fort Collins, Colorado

AUTHORS

MYRA F. BARRETT, DVM, MS
Diplomate, American College of Veterinary Radiology; Assistant Professor of Radiology, Department of Environmental and Radiological Health Sciences, Veterinary Teaching Hospital, Colorado State University, Fort Collins, Colorado

DANIEL J. BURBA, DVM
Diplomate, American College of Veterinary Surgeons; Professor of Large Animal Surgery, Department of Veterinary Clinical Sciences, School of Veterinary Medicine, Louisiana State University, Baton Rouge, Louisiana

ELIZABETH M. CHARLES, DVM, MA
Instructor and Resident in Diagnostic Imaging, College of Veterinary Medicine, Western University of Health Sciences, Temecula, California

JEAN-MARIE DENOIX, DVM, PhD
Diplomate, European College of Veterinary Diagnostic Imaging; Agrégé, Professor, Anatomy and Lameness Diagnosis in Horses, Goustranville; Université Paris-Est, Maisons-Alfort, France

DAVID D. FRISBIE, DVM, PhD
Diplomate, American College of Veterinary Surgeons, and American College of Veterinary Sports Medicine and Rehabilitation; Associate Professor, Department of Clinical Sciences, Gail Holmes Equine Orthopaedic Research Center, Colorado State University, Fort Collins, Colorado

LORRIE GASCHEN, PhD, DVM, Dr Med Vet
Diplomate, European College of Veterinary Diagnostic Imaging; Professor of Diagnostic Imaging, Department of Veterinary Clinical Sciences, School of Veterinary Medicine, Louisiana State University, Baton Rouge, Louisiana

CARTER E. JUDY, DVM
Diplomate, American College of Veterinary Surgeons; Equine Surgeon, Alamo Pintado Equine Medical Center, Los Olivos, California

DANA A. NEELIS, DVM, MS
Diplomate, American College of Veterinary Radiology; Clinical Assistant Professor, Department of Small Animal Clinical Sciences, Virginia-Maryland Regional College of Veterinary Medicine, Blacksburg, Virginia

NATHAN C. NELSON, DVM, MS
Diplomate, American College of Veterinary Radiology; Assistant Professor, Diagnostic Imaging, College of Veterinary Medicine, Michigan State University, East Lansing, Michigan

ANTHONY PEASE, DVM, MS
Diplomate, American College of Veterinary Radiology; Section Chief, Veterinary Diagnostic Imaging, College of Veterinary Medicine, Michigan State University, East Lansing, Michigan

SARAH M. PUCHALSKI, DVM
Diplomate, American College of Veterinary Radiology; Associate Professor of Diagnostic Imaging, Department of Surgical and Radiological Sciences, School of Veterinary Medicine, University of California, Davis, Davis, California

NORMAN W. RANTANEN, DVM, MS
Diplomate, American College of Veterinary Radiology; Equine Imaging Consultant, Fallbrook, California

DAVID J. REESE, DVM
Diplomate, American College of Veterinary Radiology; Assistant Professor, Diagnostic Imaging, College of Veterinary Medicine, University of Florida, Gainesville, Florida

GREGORY D. ROBERTS, DVM, MS
Diplomate, American College of Veterinary Radiology; Clinical Associate Professor, Radiology, Veterinary Clinical Sciences, Washington State University College of Veterinary Medicine, Pullman, Washington

MICHAEL ROSS, DVM
Diplomate, American College of Veterinary Surgeons; Professor, Equine Surgery, Department of Clinical Studies, New Bolton Center, University of Pennsylvania, Kennett Square, Pennsylvania

TRAVIS C. SAVERAID, DVM
Diplomate, American College of Veterinary Radiology; Owner and Consulting Radiologist, VetRadiologist LLC, St Paul, Minnesota

KURT SELBERG, MS, DVM
Assistant Professor, Diagnostic Imaging, Department of Biosciences and Diagnostic Imaging, College of Veterinary Medicine, University of Georgia, Athens, Georgia

ALEJANDRO VALDÉS-MARTÍNEZ, MVZ
Diplomate, American College of Veterinary Radiology; Assistant Professor of Diagnostic Imaging, Department of Environmental and Radiological Health Sciences, College of Veterinary Medicine and Biomedical Sciences, Colorado State University, Fort Collins, Colorado

NATASHA M. WERPY, DVM
Diplomate, American College of Veterinary Radiology; Associate Professor, Diagnostic Imaging; Small Animal Clinical Sciences, Radiology Department, College of Veterinary Medicine, University of Florida, Gainesville, Florida

MATTHEW D. WINTER, DVM
Diplomate, American College of Veterinary Radiology; Assistant Professor and Service Chief, Diagnostic Imaging, Small Animal Clinical Sciences, College of Veterinary Medicine, University of Florida, Gainesville, Florida

LISA J. ZEKAS, DVM
Diplomate, American College of Veterinary Radiology; Diplomate, American Board of Veterinary Practitioners (Equine Practice); Associate Professor, Diagnostic Imaging, College of Veterinary Medicine, The Ohio State University, Columbus, Ohio

Contents

> Tremendous growth and advancement in equine diagnostic imaging necessitates a systematic approach to the application of these modalities to lameness diagnosis. This systematic approach must include attention to the history, physical and clinical examinations, and parameters set forth by the client. It also must include an understanding of which imaging modality is most appropriate given the details of the case. This article presents a basic framework with an underlying algorithmic foundation that can be applied when selecting imaging modalities during lameness evaluation and includes case examples demonstrating application of the approach.

> As availability increases and cost decreases, digital radiograph systems become more common in equine practice. Technological advances provide an array of choices for the equine practitioner considering purchase. Two classes of systems are available: computed radiography and flat-panel systems (direct radiography). Image processing encompasses all manipulations performed on an image at acquisition and can have a profound effect on the final digital radiograph. Consideration should be given to the type of display monitor because many options are now available. The type of display monitor and the viewing environment have an effect on interpretation performance.

> The many advancements in ultrasound technology, including spatial compounding, harmonic imaging, multidimensional and extended field-of-view images, and improvements in transducer capabilities, are used to enhance the ultrasonographic examination of the equine patient. The improvements in software and hardware capabilities help overcome artifacts, improve image quality, and allow better documentation of the examination for follow-up studies. In addition, the ability of smaller, more portable machines to produce better images is ideal for the ambulatory practice setting.

Clinical indications, technical aspects, principles of image interpretation, and advantages and disadvantages of this imaging technique for the evaluation of the equine stifle joint are discussed in this article.

The usefulness of magnetic resonance (MR) imaging in the diagnosis of equine lameness is unquestionable. As with most imaging modalities, advances in technology happen quickly, and the information that can be obtained can seem limitless. An understanding of MR sequences, expected signal intensity of normal tissues, and the role of multiplanar imaging is the foundation for interpreting MR images. The rapid development of new techniques and sequences and the potential for biochemical changes to be indirectly assessed using MR spectroscopy offer possibilities for the continued development of this modality and ensure its continued application in the diagnosis of equine lameness.

The use of intravenous gadolinium contrast during equine magnetic resonance imaging (MRI) is a new technique that has been infrequently used in clinical imaging. This article describes the development of an effective contrast dose and the use of gadolinium contrast in clinical equine MRI. Gadolinium contrast improves lesion conspicuity across a broad range of lesion types. Contrast-enhanced MRI is potentially a valuable imaging tool in the assessment of the equine athlete.

The use of molecular imaging of cartilage is the next vital step in understanding, treating, and training the equine athlete. Because of the logistics of precontrast and postcontrast medium imaging, the clinical usefulness of the examination has come into question. With the large number of horses undergoing high-field magnetic resonance imaging, the use of contrast medium administration and T1 mapping or T2 imaging precontrast and postcontrast medium administration may add a limited amount of time to the scan and has the potential to provide more detailed information about the chemical composition of the articular cartilage that is not seen with routine imaging.

Magnetic resonance imaging (MRI) allows for excellent evaluation of many types of soft tissue and osseous lesions. Using MRI as a diagnostic modality can help in developing an individualized treatment protocol. Case management can include both surgical and medical intervention. Various MRI findings and associated treatment protocols are described.

Recheck magnetic resonance imaging (MRI) studies are critical to assess response to treatment and correctly determine both a horse's ability to return to exercise and an appropriate exercise program. As with any other modality, many diagnoses require additional monitoring. This principle applies to MRI despite the more significant financial investment and potential requirement for general anesthesia. This article explores the use of recheck MRIs in case management and proposes time frames for these studies based on the initial diagnosis.

VETERINARY CLINICS OF
NORTH AMERICA: EQUINE PRACTICE

THE CLINICS ARE NOW AVAILABLE ONLINE!
Access your subscription at:
www.theclinics.com

VETERINARY CLINICS OF NORTH AMERICA: EQUINE PRACTICE

Advances in Equine Dentistry

FORTHCOMING ISSUES

Apr 2013
Topics in Equine Anesthesia
Stuart Clark-Price, DVM, MS, Guest Editor

August 2013
Advances in Equine Dentistry
Jack Easley, DVM, MS, Guest Editor

December 2013
Equine Ophthalmology
Rodney Belgrave, DVM, MS, and
Anthony Yu, DVM, MS, Guest Editors

RECENT ISSUES

August 2012
Therapeutic Farriery
Stephen E. O'Grady, DVM, MRCVS, APF,
and Andrew H. Parks, VetMB, MS, MRCVS,
Guest Editors

April 2012
Ambulatory Practice
David W. Ramey, DVM, and
Mark R. Baus, DVM, Guest Editors

December 2011
Clinical Neurology
Thomas J. Divers, DVM, and
Amy L. Johnson, DVM, Guest Editors

RELATED ISSUE

Veterinary Clinics of North America: Small Animal Practice
LM 2012 (Vol. 42, No. 4)
Genetics

Preface

Advances in Equine Imaging

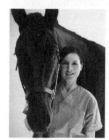 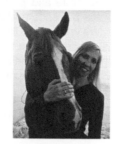

Natasha M. Werpy, DVM   Myra F. Barrett, DVM, MS
Guest Editors

Now is an exciting time to be involved with equine diagnostic imaging. Advancements in diagnostic imaging are happening at a rapid pace, and the information gained from these advancements are furthering our diagnostic capabilities and improving our patients' lives. Along with these developments comes the need for an increased understanding of the different modalities to ensure that they are used properly and to their fullest extent. In this issue of *Veterinary Clinics of North America: Equine Practice*, we strive to present the recent innovations and how they can improve your diagnostic capabilities, from radiographs and ultrasound, which are used daily in practice, to advanced imaging, which is being utilized with increased frequency.

We feel very fortunate to be involved with equine imaging, especially under the mentoring of world-renowned radiologists such as Drs Norman Rantanen and Richard Park. They have played a critical role in the evolution of radiographs and ultrasound in veterinary medicine over the past decades, which has resulted in great progress in equine practice. Similarly, we are currently experiencing a pivotal time for equine imaging with the increased availability and use of advanced imaging. Advanced imaging has added a whole new realm of diagnostic information. However, no matter what the advances, imaging information is not complete without the clinical evaluation. Furthermore, research demonstrating the relationship between imaging and the clinical conditions that we deal with in practice plays an essential role in understanding how to use imaging modalities.

We have also had the privilege to work with Dr Wayne McIlwraith, the director of the Colorado State University Gail Holmes Equine Orthopaedic Research Center, and senior scientists, Drs David Frisbie and Christopher Kawcak, and learned from their unparalleled clinical and research knowledge. For this experience we are forever grateful. This kind of partnership, between imaging specialists, clinicians, and researchers, enriches all involved and is of great benefit to our patients.

Combining expertise in diagnostic imaging and clinical assessment ensures the acquisition of appropriate images using the correct modality, allowing an accurate

Vet Clin Equine 28 (2012) xiii–xiv
http://dx.doi.org/10.1016/j.cveq.2012.09.006
0749-0739/12/$ – see front matter © 2012 Published by Elsevier Inc.

diagnosis with clinical relevance, and subsequently the best management plan for the horse. We selected authors with imaging expertise and a true understanding of the clinical relevance of their topic. We would like to sincerely thank the authors for their dedication in producing high-quality articles that combine clinical experience with current research, providing clinically accessible and pertinent information. We are grateful to John Vassallo of Elsevier for his patience and support and for providing us the opportunity to produce this issue. We would also like to thank the many others who have contributed to our educational process along the way, making this edition possible. Diagnostic imaging will continue to revolutionize veterinary medicine and improve equine practice. We can't wait to see what the next decade brings.

Natasha M. Werpy, DVM
University of Florida Veterinary Teaching Hospital
Radiology Department
2015 SW 16th Avenue
Gainesville, FL 32608, USA

Myra F. Barrett, DVM, MS
Colorado State University Veterinary Teaching Hospital
300 W. Drake
Fort Collins, CO 80523, USA

E-mail addresses:
equinedxim@yahoo.com (N.M. Werpy)
myra@colostate.edu (M.F. Barrett)

An Approach to Imaging Algorithms for Equine Lameness Diagnosis

Elizabeth M. Charles, DVM, MA[a],*,
Norman W. Rantanen, DVM, MS, DACVR[b]

KEYWORDS

- Imaging modality • Algorithms • Equine lameness

KEY POINTS

- Advances in diagnostic imaging available for the equine patient necessitate implementation of an algorithmic approach to imaging selection in lameness evaluation.
- Deciding which imaging modality is most appropriate includes assimilating information gained during the history, physical and/or clinical examination, and parameters set forth by the client.
- Every lameness situation is unique, so equine practitioners cannot rely on a "one-size-fits-all" imaging selection protocol.

INTRODUCTION

The last 15 years have seen tremendous growth and advancement in equine diagnostic imaging. Increased availability of MRI, CT, and nuclear scintigraphy, as well as technical improvements associated with digital radiography and ultrasound, give the equine practitioner a vast array of diagnostic tools to help determine the cause of lameness. With this surge in diagnostic information comes the need to better understand each of the available imaging modalities. Specifically, the equine practitioner must be able to clearly identify which imaging modality will provide the best information for lameness diagnosis given the history, physical and/or clinical examination, and parameters set forth by the client, such as budget and performance goals. Developing a systematic approach to the application of imaging modalities within the process of lameness diagnosis gives the equine practitioner a consistent method and evidence-based approach to lameness diagnosis. This process will improve patient outcomes and provide a framework to gather clinical data that can be shared with colleagues.[1]

No financial support was received for this data.
Authors have nothing to disclose.
[a] Western University of Health Sciences, College of Veterinary Medicine PO Box 38, Temecula, CA 92593, USA; [b] PO Box 2950, Fallbrook, CA 92088, USA
* Corresponding author.
E-mail address: echarles@westernu.edu

Historically, lameness evaluation has relied heavily on practitioner experience and subjective clinical impressions.[2] Improvement in imaging modalities available for use in equine patients has not changed this dramatically because localization of lameness during the clinical examination is still paramount in determining which imaging modality is most appropriate. However, advances in imaging allow for a more definitive diagnosis of lameness. The best current example of this progress is illustrated by considering lameness that originates in the foot.

Before the use of advance imaging, a right forelimb lameness that blocked to a palmar digital nerve block (PDNB) and then switched to a left forelimb lameness that was also alleviated with a PDNB was a clinical pattern attributed to "navicular disease" and was often treated with conservative therapy or neurectomy. Now, veterinarians understand that this clinical presentation could be the result of numerous types of injuries within the hoof capsule,[3,4] not just injury to the navicular bone. Many of these injuries will not respond to the traditional conservative therapy.[5] Advances in the profession have helped lead toward a more scientific, evidence-based approach to lameness, one in which synthesis of the history, clinical examination, and owner expectations and goals for the use of the horse, with diagnostic imaging findings lead to a more accurate diagnosis and appropriate treatment plan. An approach for this process using an algorithmic foundation is presented in this article.

The goal of this article is not to provide an algorithm for every possible lameness scenario. Instead, the goal is to provide a basic framework with an underlying algorithmic foundation that can be applied to choosing imaging modalities during lameness evaluation. The approach presented here is not meant to be a recipe that should be followed in every situation. Instead, it is a guideline for developing a systematic thought process and approach to selecting the appropriate imaging modality, one that takes into consideration the many nuances associated with working with horse owners and equine patients.

In a perfect world, the veterinarian could make all lameness evaluation decisions based on case-controlled studies that not only support how the clinical data should be interpreted but also which diagnostic modality is most appropriate for arriving at the correct diagnosis. The client's opinions and ideas would not come into play nor would the client's financial circumstances. Thousands of cases compiled into rigorously reviewed clinical research would support or refute the use of the available treatment options. The profession is moving toward an evidence-based approach to lameness evaluation, diagnosis, and treatment. However, every diagnostic decision the veterinarian makes is influenced by factors unrelated to the actual lameness problem, such as financial constraints. The approach presented attempts to factor in many of the influences affecting the decision-making process so the most appropriate imaging modality for the situation can be selected.

Khalil and colleagues[6] define an algorithm as "a widespread instrument for increasing efficacy and managing quality in medicine by the implementation of specified standards into a systematic, logical, evidence-based, and rational concept." In human medicine, thousands of algorithms using data collected in thousands of clinical studies have been published to aid clinicians in the delivery of appropriate care to their patients.[7] The same is not true of veterinary medicine. Although more prevalent in small animal medicine and surgery than in equine medicine and surgery, very few algorithms for equine lameness and imaging have been published.[8,9] This article uses the term algorithm loosely because there are no published data or case numbers to warrant the development of algorithms such as those published in human medicine.

As the standard of care in equine veterinary medicine continues to improve, attention to a systematic, logical, evidence-based approach to lameness and imaging is essential. The following basic outline forms the foundation of the algorithmic approach (**Fig. 1**):

1. Establish a relationship with the client.
2. Obtain a complete history.
3. Discuss expectations, goals, and financial considerations.
4. Examine the horse.
5. Localize the lameness.
6. Choose an appropriate imaging modality.
7. Revisit expectations and goals in light of initial diagnostic imaging results.
8. Further localize the lesion, if necessary.
9. Use an advanced imaging modality, if warranted.
10. Arrive at a final diagnosis.
11. Develop and implement a treatment plan.

The goal of this paper is to focus on the portions of the algorithm that pertain to choosing the appropriate imaging modality. Although it is recognized these decisions are influenced by factors seemingly unrelated to choosing the best imaging modality. For example, availability of imaging modalities within the practice area will influence which imaging modality can be chosen, as will the client's financial constraints. Thus, the history, clinical examination, expectations and goals, and localization of lameness are all important because the information gained during every step in the process will inform the decisions made with regard to imaging modality.

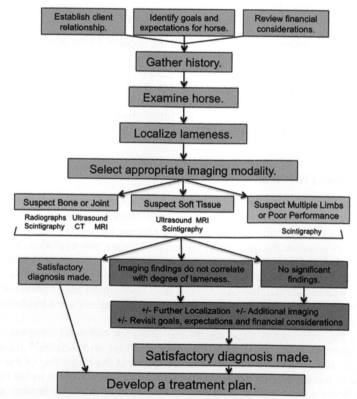

Fig. 1. Basic imaging algorithm for equine lameness diagnosis.

ESTABLISH A RELATIONSHIP WITH THE CLIENT

An effective algorithm for use in lameness and imaging does not start with the physical examination of the horse. Effective and appropriate communication with all members of the horse's team is critical and it begins with establishing a relationship.[10] Not only will such effort result in key information regarding the horse's condition, it will also eliminate confusion and unclear or unmet expectations, as well as reduce the chance of an undesirable outcome for all parties involved.

Because equine practice is so varied (eg, solo practitioner vs referral hospital vs group ambulatory practice), a one-size-fits-all approach to relationship-building and communication does not work. In equine veterinary medicine, establishing a relationship with the client can be difficult because often, it is more than just the client who is involved with the horse. Multiple scenarios are possible. The horse may just have one owner who is also responsible for all the care and training of the horse. A trainer could be involved with the owner. The owner may be an absentee owner and the trainer makes all the decisions. Or, there could be multiple owners, as is common in the racing industry, all with potentially different expectations.

To get an accurate history, understand all the expectations and future goals for the horse, and to communicate effectively about the options available for diagnostics in a lameness case, all parties must be included in the conversation in a way that allows the financially responsible person and/or party to be comfortable. Ultimately, it is the relationship with the client that will direct what the veterinarian can and cannot do from a diagnostic standpoint.

EXPECTATIONS, GOALS, FINANCIAL CONSIDERATIONS

The algorithm for working up a lameness case will depend on the client's expectations and goals (eg, broodmare expected to be sound enough to stand in the pasture vs preliminary level event horse vs grand prix jumper) as well as the client's financial resources (eg, obtain the most information for the smallest amount of expense vs no financial restrictions). Veterinarians must assimilate the client's wishes, stay within the budget, and communicate clearly and often about how the constraints of the budget are affecting the progression of the case, all while trying to arrive at a correct diagnosis.[11]

OBTAIN A COMPLETE HISTORY

When working up a complicated lameness case, obtaining a complete history is essential and can change the course of decision-making. For example, if the horse has already had diagnostic imaging, this may change the initial choice of modality, depending on whether the previously acquired images are available. A complete history includes signalment (age, sex, breed, use) and a summary of the current problem (ie, precipitating event, duration, treatments tried and response to those treatments, exacerbating activities).[12,13] Detailed information about previous medical issues or musculoskeletal injuries as well as how those issues were treated may also be important.

Because the veterinarian depends on the client for historical information, using effective communication skills is critical. Dysert, Coe, and Adams[14] have shown that failing to allow the client to voice their concerns at the beginning of the appointment leads to increased client complaints. Thus, allowing the client to tell their story about the horse's condition is paramount. This is best done by asking an open-ended question and then allowing the client to talk.[15] Veterinarians do not often choose this approach because of concerns that the client will ramble about the problem. Though veterinarians are only beginning to better understand the role of effective communication in the veterinarian-client relationship, research done in human medicine is helpful. Contrary to popular belief, the patient will often provide a succinct summary of his or her concern in less than 3 minutes.[16] Preliminary work in veterinary medicine suggests similar timeframes will hold true in veterinarian-client interactions.[17] After allowing the client the opportunity to share information, the veterinarian can then ask clarifying questions to gain better understanding. Including any other veterinarians involved with the case can shed light on the problem as well.

EXAMINE THE HORSE AND LOCALIZE THE LAMENESS

An in-depth discourse about lameness evaluation and localization is beyond the scope of this article. However, three important points should be considered here because these play a large role in determining which imaging modality to select.

First, lameness detection is a very subjective process. Research indicates that equine practitioners often differ in the interpretation of lameness evaluation performed on the same horse.[18] More specifically, when watching the same horse trot, practitioners often do not agree on which limb is the lame limb. In an effort to move toward more objective assessment of lameness, slow-motion video, force plate evaluation, and, most recently, development of the Lameness Locator Needs a registered trademark. (Equinosis, Columbia, Missouri, USA) have been implemented to increase the ability to accurately assess which limb is lame.[19,20] As lameness detection becomes more objective and accurate, correct imaging modality selection will also become easier.

Second, many of the diagnostic tests used to determine the source of pain are also subjective. Flexion tests, hoof tester evaluation, and numerous other manual manipulations used to detect and localize pain are all subject to evaluator bias and interpretation, which may or may not be accurate.[21–24] As mentioned above, as equine practitioners begin to use diagnostic tests that are objective in nature and reliably repeatable, correct imaging modality selection will become easier.

Finally, research evaluating the sensitivity and specificity of diagnostic anesthesia has revealed that absolute anatomic boundaries in the interpretation of results cannot be relied on.[25] For example, significant proximal diffusion of anesthetic along the neurovascular bundle is possible after performing a PDNB or when attempting to desensitize the palmar metacarpal nerves.[26,27] Type of anesthetic, volume of anesthetic, time following administration of the anesthetic, and the blocking technique used are all factors that need to be considered when interpreting the patient's response.[28–30]

SELECTING AN IMAGING MODALITY

The equine practitioner has numerous diagnostic imaging options when working up a lameness case. When selecting a modality, several factors must be considered. As mentioned above, the owner's goals, objectives, and financial situation all shape the direction of case management. The clinical evaluation may direct toward a modality more suited to soft tissue (ultrasound, MRI) or may put osseous injury higher on the list (radiography, CT, scintigraphy). If the patient is going to be evaluated in the field, options are limited to radiography and ultrasound. The availability of advanced imaging may affect possible options as well.

Radiography is often the first modality of choice for several reasons. It provides excellent visualization of osseous structures, is readily available, can rule out numerous differential diagnoses, and is cost-effective. Radiography not only helps rule out osseous injury but also gives the practitioner historical and baseline information about the imaged osseous structures. The downside to radiography is its inability to detect lesions unless a significant amount of pathologic change is present. It can also be difficult to identify nondisplaced fractures unless the beam is directed at precisely the angle of the fracture line.

Ultrasound is also readily available and cost-effective. Although ultrasound is generally thought of as providing excellent soft tissue images, it is also more sensitive to small, superficial osseous abnormalities than radiographs are. It is a great adjunct to radiography when an equivocal bone lesion is identified radiographically and is in a region that is accessible with ultrasound. Obtaining diagnostic images is very operator dependent. Therefore, ensuring the sonographer has adequate training and skill is essential.

Certain modalities, such as MRI and scintigraphy, can reveal multiple findings. These findings then need to be evaluated to determine which have clinical significance. In contrast to several findings from one imaging study, a lack of findings also provides important information, even though this is often seen as unrewarding and can be interpreted as a waste of money. Ruling out a diagnosis brings the veterinarian one step closer to finding the answer.

All modalities have advantages and disadvantages that should be considered and presented in the decision-making process.[31] The inherent advantages and disadvantages of each modality do not change. However, the modality that is most appropriate given all the factors in the case is what affects the selection process. What is seen as an advantage to one client (definitive diagnosis with advanced imaging) may be seen as a disadvantage another client (too expensive and does not really need a definitive answer). This complex decision-making process is demonstrated in the following case presentations. The algorithmic approach will be applied to each scenario. Key questions will be considered at each junction to help the reader better understand how to use the algorithmic approach in a real-world situation. Although the emphasis will be on questions related to selecting the best imaging modality for the situation, a brief synopsis of the first four steps in the decision tree is included.

CASE #1
Owner Goals, Expectations, and Financial Considerations

The first case is a 17-year-old Quarter Horse gelding owned by a 63-year-old widow who uses the horse mostly as a trail-riding horse, but she also does a little arena work with the horse. The horse is not ever used competitively. The owner would like to continue to use the horse as her riding horse, but if he is not able to do so comfortably and safely with minimal management and expense, she will retire him to a large grass pasture if that scenario will allow him a comfortable life. The owner is on a budget but recognizes the importance of understanding the cause of her horse's lameness. She asks to be informed about all costs as the process unfolds.

History

The horse has had a chronic right forelimb lameness that was treated with nonsteroidal antiinflammatory drugs, rest, and corrective shoeing, which allowed the horse to continue as a trail horse for approximately 6 months with minimal evidence of lameness. He presented because his lameness is no longer responsive to the conservative treatment strategy.

Lameness Examination

On examination, the horse showed a grade 3/5 right forelimb lameness when trotting in a straight line. Circling, both to the right and to the left, exacerbated the lameness. No evidence of soft tissue swelling was noted nor was the patient sensitive to application of the hoof testers to either front foot. Flexion of the right front distal limb was positive. Following PDNB, the horse was markedly improved, indicating the source of the lameness is likely in the foot, although lameness originating more proximally in the limb cannot be completely ruled out. With the right foot blocked, the horse did not show any evidence of lameness in the left forelimb.

Imaging Selection

Based on the patient's signalment and the blocking pattern, injury to one or more structures in the foot, either osseous or soft tissue in origin, is possible. Radiography is readily available and is often the preferred first-line diagnostic imaging modality. In this case, radiographs of the right front foot were within normal limits. Two options exist for this scenario. Either the lesion is not radiographically evident (early osseous change or soft tissue injury) or the lameness has not been localized correctly.

Taking into account the patient's breed (Quarter Horse), history (chronic lameness), and response to conservative therapy, a soft tissue injury within the hoof capsule or an osseous abnormality not identified on radiographs are ranked higher than improper localization of the lameness (**Fig. 2**). MRI provides superior visualization of the soft tissue structures within the hoof capsule. MRI is chosen over further localization, ultrasound, CT, or scintigraphy. The client is informed of the costs associated with MRI as well as the costs associated with continuing to treat the lameness conservatively without a specific diagnosis. She approves the MRI evaluation.

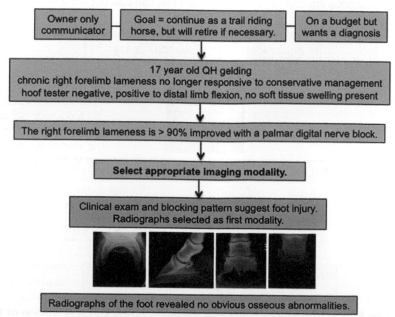

Fig. 2. Case #1 - initial evaluation and dignostic imaging.

MRI was performed and revealed a lesion in the flexor cortex of the navicular bone in the left front foot. Review of the original radiographs following lesion identification on MRI confirmed that the lesion was not identifiable on the radiographs (**Fig. 3**).

CASE #2

Owner Goals, Expectations, and Financial Considerations

The second case is a 10-year-old Warmblood (WB) gelding that is used as a 1.40 m jumper. His owner is involved with his care, but the trainer manages the horse and does most of the riding. The owner hopes the horse will continue competing at his current level successfully. There are no financial constraints in this case (**Fig. 4**).

History

The horse has had a mild, intermittent lameness over the past 2 months that has responded to short rest and 1- to 2-day treatment with antiinflammatory medication. The horse presented for an acute onset left forelimb lameness following a recent competition. The lameness was more significant than previous bouts of lameness.

Lameness Examination

On examination, the horse showed a grade 3/5 left forelimb lameness that was worse in a circle to the left. The horse was moderately positive to flexion of the left front distal limb. Following a PDNB of the left front foot, the horse was markedly improved, indicating the source of the lameness is likely in the foot. However, similar to first case, lameness originating more proximally in the limb cannot be ruled out. The horse did not show any evidence of lameness in the right forelimb with the left front foot blocked.

Imaging Selection

Radiographs are again the modality of choice because they provide excellent visualization of the osseous structures, are readily available, can rule out numerous differential

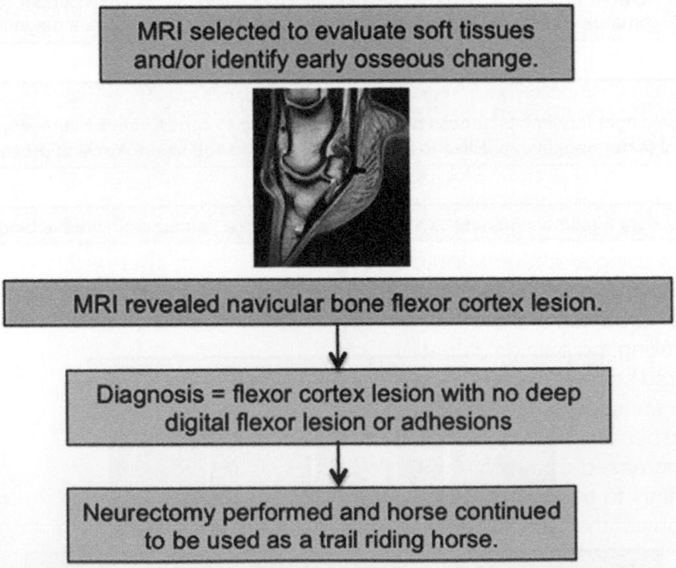

MRI selected to evaluate soft tissues and/or identify early osseous change.

MRI revealed navicular bone flexor cortex lesion.

Diagnosis = flexor cortex lesion with no deep digital flexor lesion or adhesions

Neurectomy performed and horse continued to be used as a trail riding horse.

Fig. 3. Case #1- Advanced imaging and final diagnosis. Arrow indicates location of flexor cortex lesion in the navicular bone.

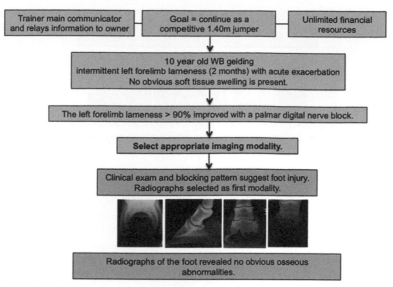

| Trainer main communicator and relays information to owner | Goal = continue as a competitive 1.40m jumper | Unlimited financial resources |

10 year old WB gelding
intermittent left forelimb lameness (2 months) with acute exacerbation
No obvious soft tissue swelling is present.

The left forelimb lameness > 90% improved with a palmar digital nerve block.

Select appropriate imaging modality.

Clinical exam and blocking pattern suggest foot injury.
Radiographs selected as first modality.

Radiographs of the foot revealed no obvious osseous abnormalities.

Fig. 4. Case #2- Initial evaluation and diagnostic imaging.

diagnoses, and are cost-effective. Radiographs of the left front foot revealed no obvious abnormalities. As in the first case, two options exist for this scenario. The lameness either has been localized appropriately and radiography does not allow the lesion to be identified in the foot (early osseous change not radiographically apparent or lesion is within the soft tissues of the foot) or the lameness is somewhere other than the foot.

The previous case had a significant amount of supporting data, in addition to the blocking pattern, to warrant MRI. The horse's breed, history, and response to treatment of the foot all pointed to the lameness being caused by injury in the foot. The data in case number two are not as cut and dry. An argument could be made that the blocking pattern, in combination with an acute or chronic presentation of a lameness that blocks to the foot, could suggest of injury to the deep digital flexor tendon at or near its insertion. It must be decided whether to trust the initial block and continue to MRI or reblock to make sure the initial localization is correct. In this case, MRI of the foot was performed. No lesions were identified. Negative radiographs coupled with a negative foot MRI make the likelihood that the lesion is in the foot unlikely. Improper localization of the lameness must now be considered.

At this juncture, two options exist. Reblocking the horse to try and further localize the lameness using a different approach than the initial examination could be considered. Alternatively, another imaging modality could also be considered. In this case, because the horse has a significant lameness and no evidence of soft tissue involvement (no swelling, no pain on palpation of the tendons and ligaments), nuclear scintigraphy (a limited scan of the front limbs instead of a complete exam of the front limbs, if money were an issue) is the most helpful modality because it will further localize the lameness, especially if osseous in nature. A limited scan of the front limbs revealed an area of increased uptake in the medial aspect of the fetlock, localizing the cause of the lameness to this region (**Fig. 5**).

Radiographs of the fetlock were within normal limits. MRI of the fetlock revealed an articular cartilage and subchondral bone defect in the medial condyle of the third metacarpal bone. Adjacent to the third metacarpal bone injury, there was diffuse fluid in the trabecular bone of the proximal phalanx.

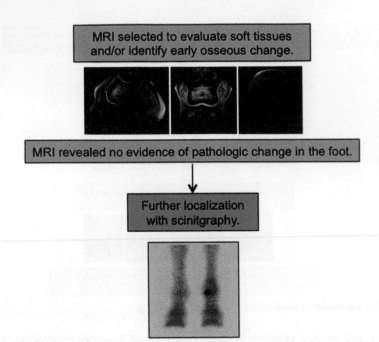

Fig. 5. Case #2- Further localization of the lameness using nuclear scinitigraphy.

This case illustrates several important points. First, diagnostic anesthesia can be very misleading. Though it is often reliable, when the blocking pattern points to a certain location but the next steps in the diagnostic plan are not supportive of a lesion in this region, another cause for the lameness must be considered. In this case, nuclear scintigraphy (instead of reblocking) led to appropriate localization of the lesion that could then be further characterized using MRI. Following MRI of the fetlock, an intraarticular fetlock joint block was performed that completely resolved the lameness, confirming that the lesion identified in the fetlock was the cause of the patient's lameness (**Fig. 6**).

Second, financial constraints were not an issue in this case. Multiple modalities were used without worrying about the overall cost to the owner. However, a limited budget would have required a different decision-making process for this case, one that may not have led to a definitive diagnosis. Instead of using scintigraphy for localization, further diagnostic blocks could have been used leading to correct localization to the fetlock, at which point MRI could have been considered because radiographs of the fetlock were inconclusive. In this case repeating the PDNB would have likely produced the same result. Therefore, a comparison of the response achieved by the PDNB to intraarticular analgesia of synovial structures that could have been affected by PDNB would have been necessary to further localize the lameness.

CASE #3
Owner Goals, Expectations, and Financial Considerations

The final case is a 10-year-old Hanoverian mare that is used predominantly as a lower-level dressage horse, but the owner also enjoys jumping. The owner would like the mare to continue competing with the hope that she will improve and move up. She is concerned about how much everything is going to cost, but is willing to do whatever is necessary as long as she is informed about the total bill at each step in the plan. She

Lesion localized to fetlock.
Fetlock MRI performed.

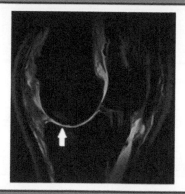

MRI revealed subchondral bone defect, MCIII

Radiographs taken post-MRI to see if
lesion could be identified radiographically.

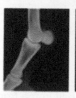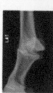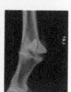

Lesion not identified radiographically.

Diagnosis = subchondral bone defect, MCIII

Horse was retired due to poor prognosis.

Fig. 6. Case #2- Advanced imaging and final diagnosis of subchondral bone defect. Arrow indicates location of subchondral bone defect and associated fluid.

informs the veterinarian that she may have to wait to do certain tests so she can save enough money to pay at the time of service (**Fig. 7**).

History

The mare has started to resist moving in a collected frame. The owner also notes that the mare's behavior has changed. The mare used to be very willing to work and is now no longer interested. The mare has also started refusing jumps.

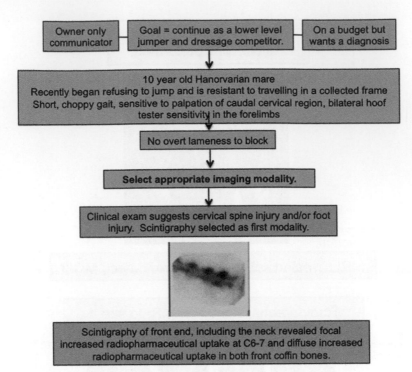

Fig. 7. Case #3- Initial evaluation and diagnostic imaging.

Lameness Examination

On examination, the horse showed a short, choppy gait in the front, though no overt lameness was appreciated. The mare was resistant to circle to the right when on the lunge line. She was also sensitive to hoof testers in both front feet as well as sensitive to palpation of the caudal neck. Her lateral cervical range of motion, subjectively assessed using the treat at the flank test, was decreased to the right when compared with the left.

Imaging Selection

Based on the clinical picture, short choppy gait in front with a resistance to bend and subjective decrease in cervical range of motion, the likelihood of two separate issues, one in the feet and one in the neck, was considered. If there was no evidence of foot pain, cervical radiographs could have been considered. If there was no evidence of cervical involvement, diagnostic analgesia of the feet could have been considered. Multiple issues coupled with the owner's report of poor performance made nuclear scintigraphy the modality of choice, specifically a front-end bone scan, including the neck.

Scintigraphic examination revealed increased radiopharmaceutical uptake in the caudal cervical facets, specifically C6-C7. Mild, diffuse increased radiopharmaceutical uptake was also seen in both front coffin bones.

Discussion with the owner led her to opt for treatment of the facet joints. Because treatment of the facet requires ultrasound guidance, facet arthrosis was confirmed when the joints were treated. Following treatment, the mare was significantly

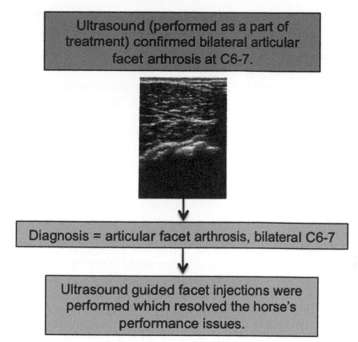

Fig. 8. Case #3 Treatment and confirmation of cervical facet arthrosis using ultrasound.

improved for approximately 8 months, at which point she began showing similar clinical signs. Treatment of the facet joints was done again with similar response (**Fig. 8**).

SUMMARY

Continued growth and advancement in equine diagnostic imaging, coupled with increased availability of advanced imaging modalities, will require equine practitioners to better understand each of the available modalities. The algorithmic approach described above gives practitioners a system for assimilating information gathered during the history, physical and/or clinical examination, and other parameters set forth by the client into an appropriate diagnostic imaging plan. This systematic approach will lead to more accurate diagnoses and improved patient outcomes.

REFERENCES

1. Johnson KA, Svirbley JR, Sriram MG, et al. Automated medial algorithms: issues for medical errors. J Am Med Inform Assoc 2002;9:S56–7.
2. Marks D. Foreward. In: Ross MW, Dyson SJ, editors. Diagnosis and management of lameness in the horse. Philadelphia: WB Saunders; 2003. p. xiii.
3. Sampson SN, Schneider RK, Gavin PR, et al. Magnetic resonance imaging findings in horses with recent onset navicular syndrome but without radiographic abnormalities. Vet Radiol Ultrasound 2009;50:339–46.
4. Dyson S, Murray R. Magnetic resonance imaging evaluation of 264 horses with foot pain: the podotrochlear apparatus, deep digital flexor tendon and collateral ligaments of the distal interphalangeal joint. Equine Vet J 2007;39:340–3.

5. Gutierrez-Nibeyro SD, White Li NA, Werpy NM. Outcome of medical treatment for horses with foot pain: 56 cases. Equine Vet J 2010;42:680–5.
6. Khalil PN, Kleespies A, Angele MK, et al. The formal requirements of algorithms and their implications in clinical medicine and quality management. Langenbecks Arch Surg 2011;396:31–40.
7. Computer-based medical algorithms: Overview and experiences. Mednet 2005, Prague, Czech Republic. December 4-8, 2005. Tech Health Care 2005;13(5): 403–5.
8. Davies C, Shell L. Common small animal medical diagnoses: an algorithmic approach. Philadelphia: WB Saunders; 2003.
9. Argyle DJ, Brearley MJ, Turek MM, editors. Decision making in small animal oncology. Ames (IO): Blackwell; 2008.
10. Kleen JL, Atkinson O, Noordhuizen JP. Communication in production animal medicine: modeling a complex interaction with the example of dairy herd health medicine. Ir Vet J 2011;64:8.
11. Shaw JR, Adams CL, Bonnett BN, et al. Veterinarian-client-patient communication during wellness appointments versus appointments related to a health problem in companion animal practice. J Am Vet Med Assoc 2008;233:1576–86.
12. Stashak TS. Examination for lameness. In: Stashak TS, editor. Adams' lameness in horses. 5th edition. Philadelphia: Lippincott, Williams and Wilkins; 2002. p. 113–83.
13. Ross MW. Anamnesis (history). In: Ross MW, Dyson SJ, editors. Diagnosis and management of lameness in the horse. Philadelphia: WB Saunders; 2003. p. 9–14.
14. Dysert LM, Coe JB, Adams CL. Analysis of solicitation of client concerns in companion animal practice. J Am Vet Med Assoc 2011;238:1609–15.
15. Cornell KK, Kopkcha M. Client-veterinarian communication: skills for client centered dialogue and shared decision making. Vet Clin North Am Small Anim Pract 2007;37:37–47.
16. Marvel MK, Epstein RM, Flowers K, et al. Soliciting the patient's agenda: have we improved? J Am Med Assoc 1999;281:283–7.
17. Shaw JR, Adams CL, Bonnett BN, et al. Use of the roter interaction analysis system to analyze veterinarian-client-patient communication in companion animal practice. J Am Vet Med Assoc 2004;225:222–9.
18. Keegan KG, Dent EV, Wilson DA, et al. Repeatability of subjective evaluation of lameness in horses. Equine Vet J 2009;41:92–7.
19. Keegan KG, MacAllister CG, Wilson DA, et al. Comparison of an inertial sensor system with a stationary force plate for evaluation of horses with bilateral forelimb lameness. Am J Vet Res 2012;73:368–74.
20. Keegan KG, Drakmer J, Yonezawa Y, et al. Assessment of repeatability of a wireless, inertial sensor-based lameness evaluation system for horses. Am J Vet Res 2011;72:1156–63.
21. Armentrout AR, Beard WL, White BJ, et al. A comparative study of proximal hindlimb flexion in horses: 5 versus 60 seconds. Equine Vet J 2012;44(4):420–4.
22. Keg PR, van Weeren PR, Back W, et al. Influence of the force applied and its period of application on the outcome of the flexion test of the distal forelimb of the horse. Vet Rec 1997;141:463–6.
23. Kearney CM, van Weeren PR, Cornelissen BP, et al. Which anatomical region determines a positive flexion test of the distal aspect of a forelimb in a nonlame horse? Equine Vet J 2010;42:547–51.
24. Busschers E, van Weeren PR. Use of the flexion test of the distal forelimb in the sound horse: repeatability and effect of age, gender, weight, height and fetlock joint range of motion. J Vet Med A Physiol Pathol Clin Med 2001;48:413–27.

25. Schumacher J, Schramme MC, Schumacher J, et al. How to perform and interpret diagnostic analgesia of the equine foot. In: Proceedings of the AAEP focus meeting on the foot. Columbus: 2009. p. 90–102.
26. Nagy A, Bodo G, Dyson SJ, et al. Diffusion of contrast medium after perineural injection of the palmar nerves: an in vivo and in vitro study. Equine Vet J 2009; 41:379–83.
27. Nagy A, Bodo G, Dyson SJ. Diffusion of contrast medium after four different techniques for analgesia of the proximal metacarpal region: an in vivo and in vitro study. Equine Vet J 2012. [Epub ahead of print].
28. Seabaugh KA, Selberg KT, Valdes-Martinez A, et al. Assessment of the tissue diffusion of anesthetic agent following administration of a low palmar nerve block in horses. J Am Vet Med Assoc 2011;239:1334–40.
29. Schumacher J, Schumacher J, Gillette R, et al. The effects of local anaesthetic solution in the navicular bursa of horses with lameness caused by distal interphalangeal joint pain. Equine Vet J 2003;35:502–5.
30. Schumacher J, Livesey L, DeGraves FJ, et al. Effect of anaesthesia of the palmar digital nerves on proximal interphalangeal joint pain in the horse. Equine Vet J 2004;36:409–14.
31. Werpy NM. Equine imaging modalities. In: 56th Annual AAEP convention proceedings. Baltimore: 2010. p. 297–306.

Digital Radiography for the Equine Practitioner
Basic Principles and Recent Advances

Nathan C. Nelson, DVM, MS[a],*, Lisa J. Zekas, DVM[b],
David J. Reese, DVM[c]

KEYWORDS

- Digital • Equine • Radiography • DICOM • Monitor

KEY POINTS

- Two types of digital radiograph systems are available (computed radiography and flat-panel systems), each with advantages and disadvantages for the equine professional.
- Consideration of digital radiograph storage and backup is important when implementing a digital radiograph system.
- Many factors influence final digital radiograph quality, including image processing, image storage format, viewing conditions, and monitor choice.

INTRODUCTION

The first digital radiography systems were introduced in the early-1980s, but the high purchase and maintenance costs, as well as large (for the time) image storage requirements, limited their adoption in the veterinary field until the early- to mid-1990s. Even then, their implementation was primarily limited to tertiary referral centers and larger teaching hospitals. In the last 10 years, however, these systems have proliferated at a rapid rate in equine practice, with an overwhelming array of digital imaging systems now available at a variety of price points.[1] The widespread availability of different systems has profound implications to the equine practitioner, and may result in confusion and anxiety for the practitioner considering purchase. Practitioners may fear a competitive disadvantage if seen as old-fashioned by relying on conventional film-screen radiography, although conventional film-screen radiography produces high-quality diagnostic images. Though the price of digital radiography systems continues to decrease, the price of market entry is still significant. Additionally, given the ongoing

[a] Diagnostic Imaging, College of Veterinary Medicine, Michigan State University, 736 Wilson Road, East Lansing, MI 48824, USA; [b] Diagnostic Imaging, College of Veterinary Medicine, The Ohio State University, 601 Vernon L. Tharp Street, Columbus, OH 43210, USA; [c] Diagnostic Imaging, College of Veterinary Medicine, University of Florida, 2015 Southwest 16th Avenue, 2015 Southwest 16th Avenue, Gainesville, FL 32611, USA
* Corresponding author.
E-mail address: nelso329@cvm.msu.edu

Vet Clin Equine 28 (2012) 483–495
http://dx.doi.org/10.1016/j.cveq.2012.08.003
0749-0739/12/$ – see front matter © 2012 Published by Elsevier Inc.
vetequine.theclinics.com

technological evolution of digital imaging systems, practitioners may have valid concerns regarding rapid equipment obsolescence or future incompatibility.

Though the cost and technological concerns are considerable, the benefits of digital radiography often outweigh these issues. Digital systems allow a wider range of radiograph exposures than conventional film-screen systems, with fewer repeated (retake) projections if the radiographic technique is incorrect. Many digital radiography systems have an integrated portable computer monitor that displays an image within seconds of exposure, allowing confirmation of proper patient positioning and exposure settings. Digital radiograph images may be manipulated after acquisition, allowing adjustment of image contrast and digital image magnification. Creating duplicate copies of digital radiographs is quick and inexpensive, allowing multiple copies of the images to be distributed to owners or for off-site backup. Digital systems reduce the upkeep costs of traditional radiography systems, eliminating the need to replenish development chemicals or to purchase and dispose of film.

As digital radiography has become more common in the equine field, many practitioners are familiar with these inherent benefits and likely will have some experience with a digital imaging system. The purpose of this article is not to restate these many benefits but, instead, to focus on the basics of digital radiography and recent advances in technology. This knowledge is pertinent to the equine professional wishing to purchase a digital radiography system or to better understand the advantages and disadvantages of their existing system. This article provides a comprehensive introduction to the technology, recent and future advancements in the technology, and how these will continue to affect equine practitioners.

OVERVIEW OF THE DIGITAL RADIOGRAPHY PROCESS

At its most basic, digital radiography involves the exposure of a reusable digital x-ray detector to create an image that is viewed on a computer monitor, eliminating the film and viewbox used with conventional radiography. The x-ray tube and peripheral x-ray equipment are largely unchanged from those systems used for conventional radiography, so replacement of these systems is not usually necessary when making the digital transition.[2]

The digital image is comprised of rows and columns of small discrete elements (called pixels), each with a particular shade of gray. The number of pixels depends on the size of the x-ray exposure (area of collimation), but is typically 1000 to 2000 rows by 1000 to 2000 columns. When viewed in total, the rows and columns of pixels create the familiar radiographic image.

After exposure of the digital receptor (plate), the image is initially sent to a computer, sometimes called the acquisition station, for processing and adjustment. These adjustments may alter the appearance of anatomic edges, adjust the contrast and shades of gray of the image, imbed annotations within the image, or crop out unwanted anatomy.[2] The image is then finalized and downloaded to another computer, often referred to as a workstation. The workstation often has a higher quality monitor, faster processor, larger storage capacity, and more capable viewing software. It is often the location where a final diagnosis is rendered. Viewing the final image solely on the acquisition computer has some disadvantages (see later discussion).

DIGITAL IMAGING SYSTEMS

The world of digital imaging is filled with acronyms. There is broad consensus in the use of CR to represent computed radiography. The acronym DR is more ambiguous. Some sources use it to represent digital radiography, which broadly encompasses all digital imaging, including CR. Others use it to represent direct radiography or digital radiography, used synonymously with flat-panel detectors (FPDs) regardless of type (direct or indirect converting).

The image receptor defines the type of radiography used. With conventional radiography, the ultimate image receptor is the x-ray film on which the final image is imprinted with the assistance of adjacent intensifying screens. With digital radiography, a reusable receptor is used. There are two general classes of digital receptor systems common in equine practice: computed radiography imaging systems and flat-panel imaging systems (**Fig. 1**).[1] Both produce a digital image, but differ in the technology used. An additional type of digital radiography system, a charge-coupled detector, is produced but cannot be used in equine practice because it requires a permanent x-ray table that is not suitable for use with horses.[3]

Computed Radiography Imaging Systems

For CR systems, the detector is a cassette that contains a receptor plate, called a photostimulable phosphor (PSP) plate. This plate temporarily stores x-ray energy as a latent image when an exposure is made. Because of this plate, CR systems are sometimes referred to as PSP systems.[1] From the exterior, the cassette is nearly identical to a cassette used in conventional film-screen radiography (**Fig. 2**). Within the cassette, however, the CR system lacks the screens and film of conventional systems, containing only the PSP.

After exposure of the CR cassette, it is placed within a digital plate reader. This reader removes the PSP from the cassette and the x-ray latent image is read out using a laser beam. Finally, the digital plate reader erases the latent image from the phosphor plate and reinserts it within the cassette for reuse. The readout step may take anywhere from 45 seconds to several minutes depending on the processor. The image is then sent to an acquisition computer for quality-control analysis and postprocessing manipulations (eg, lightening or darkening, edge enhancement).

Flat-Panel Imaging Systems

Flat-panel imaging systems were developed later than CR systems and, as a result, have more recent advances and greater promise for further development (**Fig. 3**). CR is largely a developed technology, whereas the flat-panel system is still a developing technology. Flat-panel systems represent most digital systems currently

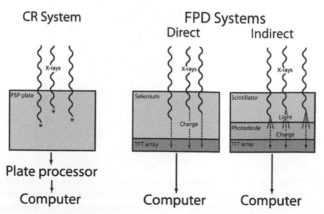

Fig. 1. CR versus direct and indirect FPDs.

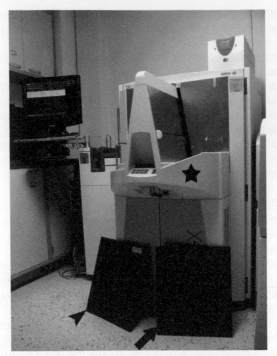

Fig. 2. CR system. Note that the PSP cassette (*arrow*) is nearly identical to a film-screen cassette (*arrowhead*). This particular CR (*star*) is a high-volume processor and, therefore, is large (smaller, tabletop and portable units are available). The acquisition computer is next to the processor.

marketed to equine professionals. Flat-panel imaging systems use an FPD, a solid-state technology that receives the x-ray energy during an exposure. An integrated readout mechanism within the detector instantly processes that energy and displays the image on a nearby computer within seconds, without any intrinsic removable parts or need of a separate plate reader.[3]

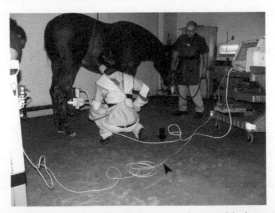

Fig. 3. Use of a FPD during hindlimb radiography. Note that a cable (*arrow*) connects the FPD to the acquisition computer on the stand. A second cable (*arrowhead*) extends from the x-ray tube to the acquisition computer; this cable sends the message to activate the FPD when an exposure is made (wireless FPD systems have eliminated the need for these cables).

The size of an FPD is not much different from a film-screen or CR cassette, but the internal structure of an FPD is not accessible. Many FPDs are slightly thicker in dimension than CR cassettes, particularly in older systems. However, the thickness of FPDs has decreased with time and the most recent are similar in dimension to CR cassettes. The internal structure of the FPD is complex, with different designs available. This complex internal structure is the source of much of the confusing sales terminology and abbreviations related to the construction of these panels.

Two major subcategories of FPD exist: direct converting and indirect converting (see **Fig. 1**).[1,3] Direct and indirect converting FPD differ in the way in which they internally convert x-ray energy into an electrical signal, which is read by the internal electronics of the plate. Indirect converting FPDs are so named because they indirectly convert x-rays to electrons. In these plates, a layer of scintillator material coats the interior surface of the plate. When x-rays strike the scintillator, visible light is produced. This light is then converted into an electrical signal by a diode underneath the scintillator. Because x-rays are converted to light before being converted into electrical signal, this type of detector is considered indirectly converting. Typically, this scintillator is either cesium iodide (CSI) or gadolinium oxysulfide (GOS). CSI is intrinsically more sensitive to x-rays than GOS (allowing lower exposure settings on the x-ray tube) and has a crystalline structure with the potential to provide greater spatial resolution. Most FPDs in the equine market today are indirect converting.

Direct converting FPDs have a layer of selenium, instead of a scintillator, immediately under the surface of the plate. When x-rays strike the selenium, electrical charge is generated directly, without converting to light, to create an electrical signal and subsequent image, hence it is direct converting.

In direct and indirect converting FPDs, a layer of transistors at the base of the plate collects the electrons generated by x-ray exposure. These transistors are arranged in a matrix of rows and columns (typically 1000 to 2000 rows and columns for a 10 × 12 in detector) and correspond to the individual pixels of the final radiographic image.[3] This layer is called a thin-film transistor array (TFT) and is made of amorphous silicon. Understanding the components of a digital radiography system can help make sense of the abbreviations and technical jargon used in naming systems. For example, if a plate is described as "amorphous silicon TFT CSI," this is an FPD because a silicon TFT layer is used and it must be indirectly converting because a CSI layer instead of selenium is used.

Recent Technological Advances

Because CR systems were developed earlier than other digital imaging systems, fewer technological developments have occurred recently relative to other imaging types and it is unlikely that many radical changes will be seen in the future. Although of primary interest for a high-volume practice, high-speed CR plate processors have been developed that use parallel laser beam stimulation to read a plate in as few as 5 seconds.[1] Dual-layer PSP plates and more sensitive PSP materials have also been developed that increase the sensitivity of the plate to x-rays. This allows a reduction in x-ray exposures to a level similar to those used in FPDs.[1,4] Most CR readers offer faster processing times and are the size of a large benchtop processor with some larger, freestanding units available. In addition, portable (<40 lb) point-of-service CR readers have been developed that are appropriate for use in the field.[1]

Because the technology is relatively new, there have been many recent advances in FPD technology. Perhaps the largest and most recent innovation is the introduction of wireless technology. These systems contain a rechargeable battery within the imaging panel, as well as a wireless transmitter. After the x-ray exposure, the imaging plate transmits the image to the computer for review. Several wireless plates are on the market; it is likely this technology will continue to become more popular. As this article goes to press, most wireless imaging panels are capable of acquiring hundreds of images before the need to recharge, with a complete recharging time of several hours. Wireless image transfer is relatively rapid, with transfer times of several seconds. When combined with new battery-powered x-ray generators, the equine professional can now acquire digital images in the field, without any of the hassles caused by cabling. Another innovation using FPD technology includes incorporating the monitor for reviewing images into the housing of the portable x-ray generator.

Direct converting FPDs are relatively new to the veterinary market compared with indirect converting FPDs. Although there are technical arguments on the pros and cons of these technologies, they are largely similar in performance. There is no clear answer to the question whether direct or indirect FPDs are superior.[1] Each has theoretical advantages and disadvantages, but they are equally effective in producing images of extremely high quality and sensitivity to x-ray exposure.[5]

Choosing an Image Detector

A variety of digital radiography receptor systems are now readily available to the equine practitioner (**Table 1**). These systems differ in their fundamental construction and capabilities, but the ultimate output is a digital radiographic image. A common question when faced with the extensive array of imaging systems on the market is "which one should I buy?" Unfortunately, there is no one right answer. The decision will largely depend on the intended purpose, frequency of use, and price.

The first decision to be made is whether a CR system or FPD will be purchased. Although most digital imaging systems marketed to the equine professional are flat-panel systems, CR systems are often an affordable choice for the practitioner wishing to enter the digital radiography market. At this time, there is not a best choice between CR and FPD; it depends on the study being performed, image quality, system cost, portability, image handling, and service and maintenance costs.[5] The intended application is of utmost importance.[5] The major disadvantage of the CR system for the equine professional is the lack of processor portability for most systems, which require that cassettes exposed in the field be returned to the practice for development and processing.[1] Additionally, CR cassettes are susceptible to scatter x-ray exposure as with conventional film-screen systems.

From an image quality standpoint, both CR and digital radiography systems produce high-quality images that are similar in image contrast and spatial resolution. Traditionally CR systems have had lower detection efficiency for x-rays than FPDs. A low detection efficient means higher x-ray exposures are required, but newer CR systems have narrowed or eliminated this advantage.[1]

CR systems have some advantages to the equine professional. Because CR is a developed technology, many high quality systems are available at affordable prices and often have a lower initial investment cost.[1] The CR cassettes are nearly identical to film-screen cassettes. They are compatible with film-holding devices and have similar functional use. Certain CR systems are able to process a variety of plate sizes. Therefore, large cassettes (14 in × 17 in, such as used for thoracic radiography) and smaller cassettes (such as those for intraoral radiography) may be used with the same digital processor. CR cassettes are also relatively inexpensive. This allows the purchase of additional cassettes. Therefore, the loss or damage of a cassette is less limiting than if an FPD is damaged. In contrast to a CR system, damage to an FPD can render the system unusable.

A major advantage of CR systems over FPD has been the ease of cassette position and handling, without the need of cables to connect the x-ray generator and FPD to an

Table 1
Specifications of various digital radiography systems offered by veterinary vendors

Vendor	Model Name	Direct or Indirect	Scintillator (If Indirect)	Tethered or Wireless-Imaging Plate	Plate Dimensions	Imaging Area	Reported Pixel Pitch (microns)	Plate Manufacturer or Model
Sound-Eklin	Mark 1114cw	Indirect	CSI	Wireless	14 in w × 15 in h × 0.9 in d	10.8 in × 13.8 in	125	Canon CXDI-80C (Canon USA, Inc, NY, USA)
Sound-Eklin	Mark 1210c	Indirect	CSI	Tethered	14 in w × 15 in h × 0.9 in d	10 in × 12 in	127	Vatech Xmaru (Vatech America, Secaucus, NJ, USA)
Sound-Eklin	Tour cSeries 1109C	Indirect	CSI	Tethered	14 in w × 15 in h × 0.9 in d	9 in × 11 in	160	Canon CXDI-60C (Canon USA, Inc, NY, USA)
Sound-Eklin	Tour eSeries 1008G	Indirect	GOS	Tethered	9 in w × 15 in h × 1 in d	8 in × 11 in	127	Varian 2520e+ (Varian Medical Systems, Palo Alto, CA, USA)
Sound-Eklin	Mark IIG	Indirect	GOS	Tethered	14 in w × 15 in h × 0.9 in d	9 in × 11 in	160	Canon CXDI-60G (Canon USA, Inc, NY, USA)
Universal	MyRad 60	Indirect	GOS	Tethered	14 in w × 15 in h × 0.9 in d	9 in × 11 in	160	Canon CXDI-60G (Canon USA, Inc, NY, USA)
Universal	UI 80	Indirect	CSI	Wireless	14 in w × 15 in h × 0.9 in d	10.8 in × 13.8 in	125	Canon CXDI-80C (Canon USA, Inc, NY, USA)
Vetel	Explorer series 60C/60G	Indirect	CSI or GOS	Tethered	14 in w × 15 in h × 0.9 in d	9 in × 11 in	160	Canon CXDI 60G or 60C (Canon USA, Inc, NY, USA)
Vetel	Explorer series 80C	Indirect	CSI	Wireless	14 in w × 15 in h × 0.9 in d	10.8 in × 13.8 in	125	Canon CXDI-80C (Canon USA, Inc, NY, USA)
Vetel	Envision series 1210C	Indirect	CSI	Tethered	16.6 in × 15.9 in × 0.9 in	10 in × 12 in	127	Vatech Xmaru (Vatech America, Secaucus, NJ, USA)
Idexx	Equiview	Direct	Not applicable	Tethered	17 in h × 13 in w × 0.9 in d	8 in × 10 in	129	DRTech (DRTech Co, Ltd, Seongnam, South Korea)
Cuattro	UnoEQ 1012	Indirect	CSI	Tethered	16.6 in × 15.9 in × 0.9 in	10 in × 12 in	127	Vatech Xmaru (Vatech America, Secaucus, NJ, USA)
Raymax	Flash Ray DR	Indirect	CSI	Tethered	16.6 in × 15.9 in × 0.9 in	10 in × 12 in	127	Vatech Xmaru (Vatech America, Secaucus, NJ, USA)

Only small size plates. Many vendors offer larger 14 in × 17 in footprints, which are not listed.
Abbreviations: d, depth; h, height; w, width.

imaging computer. Furthermore, it is not necessary to bring a computer into the field. The introduction of wireless FPD systems has greatly reduced or eliminated the portability issue.

Spatial resolution is a characteristic that may be compared between digital systems. Spatial resolution is the ability to separate two closely spaced objects on a digital image (ie, the ability to see small objects). The spatial resolution of digital systems is currently less than conventional screen-film technology, but this divide will likely lessen as technology improves.[6] The smaller the pixel of a digital image, the better the resolution. A pixel size smaller than 200 microns is recommended; most digital radiography systems on the market are capable of producing images with pixels between 130 and 160 microns. Although smaller pixel size is desirable, this should not be the only characteristic used to choose a system. There are many factors that determine the quality of a digital radiograph, including image processing and the shades of gray captured by the machine.

When assessing digital radiography systems before purchase, the most challenging images to achieve should be evaluated. In equine practice this includes the skyline view of the navicular bone, cranial-caudal of the stifle, and a lateral image of the caudal neck.

DIGITAL IMAGE PROCESSING

With conventional screen-film radiography, the appearance of the radiograph cannot be altered after film has passed through the processor. In comparison, a great advantage of digital radiography is the ability to use image processing to enhance the resulting image. Image processing is a broad term that is typically applied to all digital processes performed on an image by the detector itself and before the study is closed in final form on the acquisition device.[7] Once the final image is sent to the viewing station, some transient manipulation of the image is possible (such as the alteration of display contrast). This is broadly termed postprocessing.[7] Image processing is a broad topic and a complete review of processing principles is beyond the scope of this article. The importance of image processing may be underappreciated and, if improper processing parameters are chosen, poor quality images will be produced that obscure diagnostically relevant features.[8] Given the complexity of image processing, proper initial setup of processing protocols on the radiographic acquisition device is important.

The unprocessed, raw images generated by digital systems bear little resemblance to the final processed radiograph. Manipulation of images is necessary to improve contrast, optimize spatial resolution, and resemble what is typically considered a radiograph.[7] Although image processing software is generally similar, each manufacturer may apply algorithms, many of which are proprietary, to optimize image quality. This may result in very different appearing images between manufacturers.[6,9]

Most image processing occurs on the acquisition computer. This image processing software is usually bundled with the detector and replacement by other software is not possible.[9] Edge enhancement algorithms may be applied which result in emphasis or de-emphasis of anatomic margins, but can result in edge artifacts. Other image processing algorithms and look-up tables, which greatly alter the contrast and latitude (shades of gray) of the image, are applied by the acquisition computer.[2] If improperly applied, these manipulations may have a destructive effect on the image, causing artifacts that result in loss of anatomy (termed clipping).[10]

Once the raw digital image has been processed at the acquisition station, the final image may then be sent to a viewing station or to a teleradiology service.[7] Postprocessing image manipulation may be applied at the viewing station, but these manipulations are typically transient. Most commonly, radiograph viewing software allows control of image contrast and brightness (termed windowing and leveling). This does not result in alteration of the original stored image. However, manipulation of the window and level cannot overcome severe inadequacies in the exposure. Although this step may make the displayed image more pleasing to the viewer, if image clipping has occurred no amount of adjustment by viewing software will retrieve this information.[10]

DIGITAL IMAGE FORMAT AND STORAGE

All digital images, whether produced by digital radiograph systems or digital cameras, are stored on a computer using a particular format. There are many imaging formats in use, including JPEG (Joint Photographic Experts Group) and TIFF (tagged image file format), which are primarily used for photography or images on the web.[11] With the advent of digital radiography, it became clear that these formats were insufficient for medical use, given the need for standardization and inclusion of other medical information with the images. Digital radiography vendors initially circumvented this problem by developing different proprietary image formats, unique to each company. This was disadvantageous to the practitioner because it resulted in significant limitation. Competing technologies could not be used for image storage or interconnectivity transfer.[12] In the early 1980s, major manufacturers, working with the American College of Radiology, electronics experts, and other professional societies, developed the Digital Imaging and Communications in Medicine (DICOM) format, the complete version of which is known as the DICOM 3.0 Standard.[11]

The DICOM 3.0 Standard is a nonproprietary imaging format that defines the form and flow of electronic messages that convey imaging data between computers.[13] It serves as a storage, imaging, and data messaging standard for all types of imaging data (eg, ultrasound, MRI, endoscopy).[13] This common storage format for all vendors helps predict interoperability of imaging and storage devices.[14] It should be noted, however, that DICOM conformance is completely voluntary and there is no enforcement or testing body.[12] As a practical aside, the term DICOM is often used to refer to the image storage format when sending images.

Familiarity with DICOM format is necessary for the equine practitioner when considering the purchase of an imaging system. Because the DICOM standard is extensive, including imaging formats as well as computer connectivity and storage information, a document is required with each DICOM implementation. This document is called the DICOM Conformance Statement and details which parts of the DICOM standard are supported.[12] Any vendor providing a digital imaging system should provide this statement, particularly if other imaging components (such as dedicated computer for image storage) are to be used. DICOM conformance statements are often lengthy and contain terminology that may require interpretation by information technology professionals. Practitioners purchasing a digital system should not expect a plug and play image network setup.[13] If multiple imaging systems and computer storage devices are to be used, vendors should work with the practitioner to either demonstrate satisfactory interconnectivity before purchase or confirm interconnectivity after purchase.

Teleradiology involves the electronic transmission of digital images and other medical information to another medical professional, with such services growing at a rapid rate in the last 10 years.[15] Teleradiology provides many advantages to the equine practitioner, particularly in remote or rural locations when expedient image review is desired. Many imaging equipment vendors now are also associated with teleradiology services and may help coordinate or setup these services. If digital radiographs are to be sent to a teleradiology service or for a second opinion, it is important that the proper image format (ie, DICOM) is sent. Many digital radiography workstations export images in a JPEG format by default, instead of a DICOM format. JPEG images use lossy compression resulting in a smaller file size and an irreversible loss of imaging data.[15] These images can be easily emailed but have decreased quality and the potential for misdiagnosis.[15] Because they do not follow the DICOM format, JPEG images may not be compatible with other image-viewing software programs. JPEG images also prevent the same extent of the alterations (eg, window or level, contrast adjustment) provided by DICOM images.[15] Finally, DICOM images have embedded patient demographic information and information about image acquisition, removing ambiguity regarding the images should legal issues later arise.[13] For these reasons, the American College of Veterinary Radiology recommends that DICOM format be adopted for all teleradiology applications, with digital systems able to send DICOM images to a remote computer for evaluation.[16] Many teleradiology services can automatically download DICOM images from a practice for interpretation, removing the time-consuming step of manually exporting images and sending them through email or as a CD via the postal service.

DICOM images are a part of the medical record. Given the importance of these images, digital image storage is an important consideration for the equine practitioner. Ideally, DICOM images should be stored in a secure location with backup capabilities.[17] Legal requirements regarding veterinary image archiving differ between locations and regulatory bodies, so knowledge and adherence to local regulations are important.[18] When digital radiographs are initially captured, a copy is typically stored on the acquisition computer. Although this provides easily accessible local image storage, like any computer these devices may fail. Therefore, at least one backup copy is recommended.[17] Given the relatively large size of DICOM images, it is fortunate that many reasonably priced storage and backup solutions are available, the choice of which can be tailored to the needs of the practitioner.

Writable media such as CDs, DVDs, and Blu-ray discs are acceptable means of image backup storage in the case of primary storage failure. They are robust, inexpensive, and copies are easily made. External hard drives may also be used for backup, with prices that have greatly decreased in recent years. With such methods, a member of the practice must be responsible for maintaining the backup system (periodic backup is easily neglected). It is also recommended that backup copies be periodically removed to an offsite location for secure disaster recovery.

Offsite, third party image storage (cloud storage) is now a viable option for many practices. For a fee, companies offering this service will store digital radiographs computers, transferred to them via the Internet, on their own. In many cases, radiographic imaging systems can be configured to automatically upload images to these remote servers whenever Internet access is available. The initial cost of these services is often less than on-site backup computer systems because additional hardware or technical support time is not necessary. However, over many years, the cost of these services may be more than on-site backup options.[17] Because the cost of storage and Internet bandwidth decreases, Internet image backup will likely become more popular in the future.

IMAGE DISPLAY

When an imaging system is considered for purchase, much time may be spent comparing various system specifications between vendors. However, comparison of monitors included with these systems may be neglected. With digital radiography, the imaging chain has four steps: image acquisition, processing, archiving, and display. The performance of a system depends on all four steps.[19] The quality of a digital image is limited by the weakest link of this chain and the superior capabilities of the best imaging system will not be evident if displayed on a subpar monitor.[19]

Many advances in monitor design have been seen in the last 10 to 20 years, resulting in an array of choices to the equine practitioner. Liquid crystal displays (LCD) are flat-panel monitors and have largely replaced older style cathode ray tube monitors. When contemplating purchase of a display, the first decision is whether to choose a medical-grade monitor or a consumer-grade LCD monitor. Medical-grade monitors are designed specifically for viewing digital medical images and are available only from specialized vendors, whereas consumer-grade monitors are general-purpose monitors similar to those in electronics stores. Medical-grade LCD monitors are significantly more expensive than are consumer-grade monitors, exceeding their price by a factor of 10 or more, limiting their use in veterinary medicine.[19] Medical-grade monitors are either monochrome (ie, grayscale display only) or color, and are the standard in human medical imaging.[20] Medical-grade monitors are a higher quality product, with more rigorous testing and development, and better longevity, luminosity, and spatial resolution than off-the-shelf monitors.[21]

Luminance and spatial resolution are two key properties that define the performance of a monitor. Luminance, the brightness of the monitor, is measured in candelas per meter squared (cd/m2). Although no standards have been established in veterinary medicine, the American College of Radiology standards set a required level of at least 171 cd/m^2. However, most sources recommend a brightness of 300 to 400 cd/m^2 for diagnostic use.[22,23] Higher luminance increases perceived image quality.[24] By their nature, LCD monitors dim over time. Although high-quality consumer-grade monitors initially have adequate luminosity for diagnostic purposes, medical-grade monitors are capable of achieving higher luminosity levels, helping to offset normal age-related luminosity loss.[21] Additionally, medical-grade monitors typically include software that automatically adjusts for optimal luminance. In contrast, few consumer-grade monitors come with this software.[25]

Spatial resolution is another major consideration when comparing monitors. Monitors with higher spatial resolution contain more display pixels in a given area, resulting in the ability to visualize smaller objects. Spatial resolution is measured in megapixels (MPs), with higher numbers containing more pixels. Most medical-grade monitors contain 2 to 5 MPs.[20] If a lower spatial resolution monitor is chosen, its limitations can be overcome by digitally magnifying the image or zooming in. However, this added step will lengthen the time required to evaluate the radiograph.[19]

Regardless of the display, viewing performance is diminished significantly if monitors are used in a bright environment (eg, outdoor viewing or most barns). Control of ambient light is important for accurate interpretation, with significantly more effect on lower luminance monitors.[24,26] Higher ambient light levels also contribute to eyestrain, fatigue, and significantly decreased interpretation accuracy.[27] It is the authors' opinion that caution should be used when interpreting radiographs in a suboptimal environment, particularly if a lower quality monitor (eg, those included with many flat-panel devices) is used for diagnosis. Although medical-grade, grayscale monitors are clearly the superior monitor type for viewing radiographs their formidable price may preclude purchase. Therefore, high-quality color monitors are often sufficient for clinical purposes if care is taken to fully evaluate each image in the proper viewing environment, using magnification or other viewing tools included with viewing software packages.

SUMMARY

Digital radiography has undergone many developments since its inception nearly 30 years ago, with incremental improvements in technology likely to continue. Despite providing many advantages to the equine practitioner, digital radiography can offer a bewildering array of technologies. When evaluating a new system, characteristics of each component (ie, acquisition technology, image processing, archive and storage, and display monitor) may be evaluated separately. However, the system should also be evaluated as a sum of its parts. By witnessing a system in action or seeing examples of images produced in the field, a practitioner may be satisfied that a particular imaging system will suit his or her needs.

REFERENCES

1. Seibert JA. Digital radiography: the bottom line comparison of CR and DR technology. Appl Radiol 2009;38:21.
2. Mattoon JS. Digital radiography. Vet Comp Orthop Traumatol 2006;19:123.
3. Widmer WR. Acquisition hardware for digital imaging. Vet Radiol Ultrasound 2008;49:S2.
4. Seibert JA. Advances in computed radiography: dual-side readout. J Am Coll Radiol 2010;7:154.
5. Seibert JA. Considerations for selecting a digital radiography system. J Am Coll Radiol 2005;2:287.
6. Krupinski EA, Williams MB, Andriole K, et al. Digital radiography image quality: image processing and display. J Am Coll Radiol 2007;4:389.
7. Lo WY, Puchalski SM. Digital image processing. Vet Radiol Ultrasound 2008;49:S42.
8. Prokop M, Schaefer-Prokop CM. Digital image processing. Eur Radiol 1997; 7(Suppl 3):S73.
9. Korner M, Weber CH, Wirth S, et al. Advances in digital radiography: physical principles and system overview. Radiographics 2007;27:675.
10. Drost WT, Reese DJ, Hornof WJ. Digital radiography artifacts. Vet Radiol Ultrasound 2008;49:S48.
11. Gibaud B. The quest for standards in medical imaging. Eur J Radiol 2011;78:190.
12. Wright MA, Ballance D, Robertson ID, et al. Introduction to DICOM for the practicing veterinarian. Vet Radiol Ultrasound 2008;49:S14.
13. Bidgood WD Jr, Horii SC, Prior FW, et al. Understanding and using DICOM, the data interchange standard for biomedical imaging. J Am Med Inform Assoc 1997;4:199.
14. Kahn CE, Carrino JA, Flynn MJ, et al. DICOM and Radiology: past, present, and future. J Am Coll Radiol 2007;4:652.
15. Poteet BA. Veterinary teleradiology. Vet Radiol Ultrasound 2008;49:S33.
16. American College of Veterinary Radiology Teleradiology Guidelines; American College of Veterinary Radiology Website. Available at: http://www.acvr.org/page/teleradiology-guidelines. Accessed on January 10, 2012.
17. Wallack S. Digital image storage. Vet Radiol Ultrasound 2008;49:S37.
18. Robertson ID, Saveraid T. Hospital, radiology, and picture archiving and communication systems. Vet Radiol Ultrasound 2008;49:S19.
19. Ludewig E, Boeltzig C, Gabler K, et al. Display quality of different monitors in feline digital radiography. Vet Radiol Ultrasound 2011;52:1.
20. Puchalski SM. Image display. Vet Radiol Ultrasound 2008;49:S9.
21. Diiulio R. An eye on monitors: color is the biggest trend in medical monitors today and the costs may surprise you, but size and grade are also receiving attention. Imaging Economics 2010; 23:30.
22. ACR Technical Standard for Electronic Practice of Medical Imaging; American College of Veterinary Radiology Website. Available at: http://www.acr.org/SecondaryMainMenuCategories/quality_safety/guidelines/med_phys/Electronic_Practice.pdf. Accessed on January 10, 2012.

23. Sorantin E. Soft-copy display and reading: what the radiologist should know in the digital era. Pediatr Radiol 2008;38:1276.
24. Wang J, Langer S. A brief review of human perception factors in digital displays for picture archiving and communications systems. J Digit Imaging 1997;10:158.
25. Krupinski EA. Medical grade vs off-the-shelf color displays: influence on observer performance and visual search. J Digit Imaging 2009;22:363.
26. Ricke J, Hanninen EL, Zielinski C, et al. Shortcomings of low-cost imaging systems for viewing computed radiographs. Comput Med Imaging Graph 2000; 24:25.
27. Siddiqui KM, Chia S, Knight N, et al. Design and ergonomic considerations for the filmless environment. J Am Coll Radiol 2006;3:456.

Advances in Equine Ultrasonography

Dana A. Neelis, DVM, MS[a],*, Gregory D. Roberts, DVM, MS[b]

KEYWORDS

- Equine • Ultrasonography • Spatial compounding • Harmonics • Panoramic

KEY POINTS

- Recent advancements in ultrasound technology and software applications provide valuable tools for imaging of the equine patient.
- Alteration of the field of view is a simple method for visualizing larger structures such as the suspensory ligament.
- Harmonic imaging is useful for improving resolution of the image, particularly in the mid field.
- Spatial compounding reduces the dependence on beam angle, although it can create temporal artifacts.
- Documentation of the examination can now be performed in a multitude of ways (ie, cine loops, 3-dimensional, extended field-of-view images), allowing for better follow-up examinations and depiction of the abnormality to owners and students.

INTRODUCTION

Ultrasonography is a widely available, relatively inexpensive, and safe imaging modality commonly used in equine practice for the diagnosis of cardiac, respiratory, gastrointestinal, urinary, musculoskeletal, and reproductive disorders. Although ultrasonography is very useful, it does have some limitations in the ability to visualize certain anatomic areas and lesion types. In addition, ultrasonography is user dependent, and the ability to obtain and accurately interpret diagnostic images is a learned skill that comes with experience. Learning how to properly manipulate the controls, including the gain settings, focal zones, depth, and frequency, is key to obtaining a quality image and being confident in the ultrasonographic diagnosis. The manual

The authors have nothing to disclose.
[a] Department of Small Animal Clinical Sciences, Virginia-Maryland Regional College of Veterinary Medicine, Duck Pond Drive (0442), Blacksburg, VA 24061, USA; [b] Radiology, Veterinary Clinical Sciences, Washington State University College of Veterinary Medicine, PO Box 647010, Pullman, WA 99164-7010, USA
* Corresponding author.
E-mail address: dneelis@vt.edu

Vet Clin Equine 28 (2012) 497–506
http://dx.doi.org/10.1016/j.cveq.2012.08.001
0749-0739/12/$ – see front matter © 2012 Elsevier Inc. All rights reserved.

dexterity needed to manipulate the transducer in an optimal position relative to the structure of interest is an acquired skill. Although advanced imaging, such as computed tomography (CT) and magnetic resonance imaging (MRI), are now widely available for musculoskeletal imaging and are less user dependent, these modalities may require general anesthesia. With ultrasonography, multiple sequential examinations can be obtained without the expense and risk of general anesthesia associated with advanced imaging, making it a particularly attractive modality for equine practice. Therefore, practitioners need to be aware of and understand the advancements in ultrasound technology that are constantly being developed to help increase the diagnostic yield and overcome some of the limitations.

ULTRASOUND MACHINE ADVANCEMENTS

The resolution and detail of images obtained with ultrasound machines has greatly improved over the past 10 years owing to advancements in software applications, computer hardware, and development of high-resolution and broadband transducers. Even small, portable machines can now produce images that rival the larger machines used in a hospital setting, which is of particular importance to the ambulatory equine practitioner. Some systems have also developed ways whereby the images can be processed after acquisition, including making measurements and adjusting gain. This postprocessing is helpful when performing an examination in less than ideal circumstances (ie, poorly lit barn, outside, impatient horse).[1]

FIELD OF VIEW

The majority of musculoskeletal imaging in equine practice is performed with a linear transducer. This type of transducer produces a rectangular scan plane (**Fig. 1**A) approximately 4 to 5 cm in width. Some anatomic structures, such as the tendons and ligaments along the palmar/plantar metacarpus/metatarsus, cannot be fully visualized with the rectangular field of view in the transverse plane. Therefore, the transducer has to be moved medially and laterally across the leg to fully evaluate all of the anatomy, particularly when evaluating the suspensory ligament in the hindlimb.[2] Utilization of a trapezoidal field of view (**Fig. 1**B) is useful to better visualize the full extent of these structures, especially in the mid to far fields of the image. The field

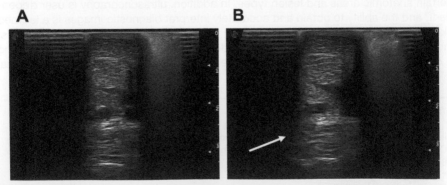

Fig. 1. Transverse images of the mid-metacarpus (lateral is to the left of the images). (*A*) Normal rectangular field of view. Notice the straight lateral margins of the field. (*B*) Trapezoidal field of view. The suspensory ligament (*arrow*) appears larger than in the rectangular field of view, as more of the ligament is able to be visualized.

of view can be easily switched from trapezoidal to linear with the push of a button on most machines. The trapezoidal function helps evaluate tendons/ligaments in the transverse plane or short axis. However, when viewing these structures in the sagittal plane or long axis, the trapezoidal field of view should not be used because it distorts the normal fiber pattern (**Fig. 2**).

HARMONICS

Harmonic imaging (**Fig. 3**) can potentially improve spatial and contrast resolution and decrease artifacts in ultrasonographic images.[3] Ultrasound pulses a sound wave at a designated frequency into tissue. The shape of the sound waveform is distorted as it propagates through different tissues, which generates echoes of multiple different frequencies. The generated frequencies are called harmonics. With harmonic imaging, the ultrasound machine processes the echoes as they return to the transducer. Typically the echoes that are allowed to pass and be processed are twice the original frequency, while unwanted frequencies are removed. The filtering of the unwanted frequencies is what effectively reduces the image noise.

Harmonic imaging is best suited for evaluation of structures in the mid field. Unfortunately, harmonic imaging does not work well for structures in the near field, as the sound wave has to interact with a sufficient amount of tissue to create a harmonic frequency, and structures in the far field are difficult to adequately visualize owing to attenuation.[1]

COMPOUND IMAGING

Compound imaging has also been used to help improve the ultrasonographic image. Spatial compound imaging is the creation of an image by averaging frames from multiple scan lines that are being steered in different directions (**Fig. 4**). The information is collected and averaged or compounded together from several different angles without having to move the transducer. Compound imaging improves the ultrasonographic image by reducing artifacts (ie, speckle, clutter), smoothing the image, improving margin definition, and allowing visualization of structures deep to highly attenuating structures (**Fig. 5**).[4] It also decreases the dependence on beam angle, known as the anisotropic effect, which is helpful in musculoskeletal imaging because

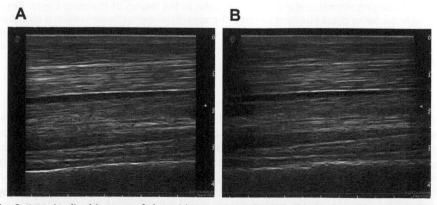

Fig. 2. Longitudinal images of the mid-metacarpus (proximal is to the left of the images). (*A*) Normal rectangular field of view. (*B*) Trapezoidal field of view. Note the distortion of the tendon and ligament fibers proximally and distally, near the periphery of the image.

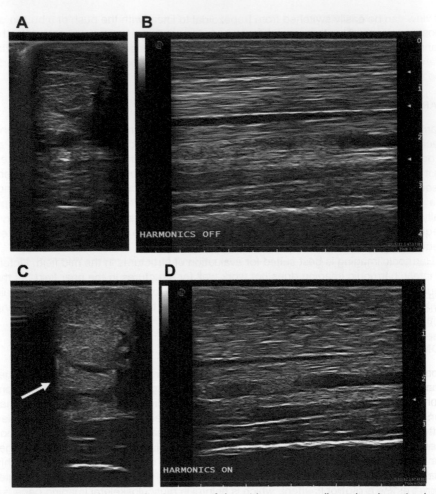

Fig. 3. Transverse and longitudinal images of the mid-metacarpus (lateral and proximal are to the left of the images). (*A, B*) Harmonics are turned off. (*C, D*) Harmonics are turned on. Harmonic imaging is most useful for the mid field, in the region of the deep digital flexor tendon and inferior check ligament (*arrow*). The superficial digital flexor tendon is indistinct because it does not produce sufficient echoes at the harmonic frequency. The echoes from the suspensory ligament are being attenuated, thus creating a very hypoechoic, poorly visualized ligament.

the transducer has to be completely perpendicular to the tendon/ligament fibers to obtain a good-quality image (**Fig. 6**A). If the transducer is not perpendicular to the fibers, areas within the tendon/ligament become more hypoechoic and may be confused with lesions (**Fig. 6**B). With compound imaging, at least one of the scan lines is usually perpendicular to the tendon or ligament fibers, so less transducer movement is required. Compound imaging is especially helpful when a tendon or ligament is traveling over a curved surface, such as in the shoulder, or when the fibers are coursing obliquely (ie, oblique distal sesamoidean ligament). One of the problems with compound imaging is that there is a decrease in temporal resolution, meaning that the image can be blurry if any patient motion is present. In addition, acoustic

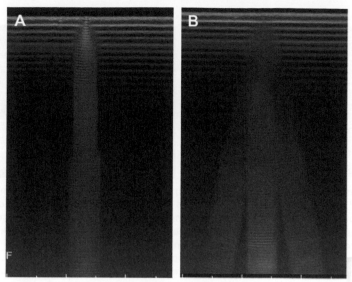

Fig. 4. Linear transducer images obtained by placing a needle transversely across the transducer. (*A*) The ultrasound beam is steered in one direction when compounding is turned off. (*B*) Compounding is turned on, and the different viewing angles from the same crystals in the transducer can be visualized.

shadowing (the dark shadow visualized deep to a strongly attenuating structure) is less evident in compound imaging; therefore, using both compound imaging and conventional imaging during an examination is recommended.[4]

Still-frame ultrasonographic images have been, and are still, the mainstay for documentation of an examination. Previously, an image was limited by the size of an individual frame from the transducer. Nowadays more informative panoramic images can be created that demonstrate the full extent of the damaged area, including the association with adjacent structures or anatomic landmarks.[3,5,6] Static B-mode scanners from the 1980s did not have the problem of the limited field of view that is encountered by the more current scanners; however, they relied on awkward, bulky sensors or

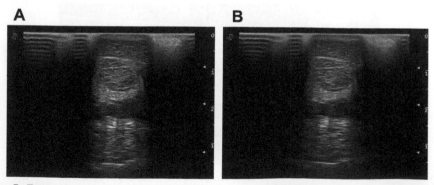

Fig. 5. Transverse images of the mid-metacarpus (lateral is to the left of the images). (*A*) Compounding is turned off. (*B*) Compounding is turned on. This image is much smoother in appearance when compared with A.

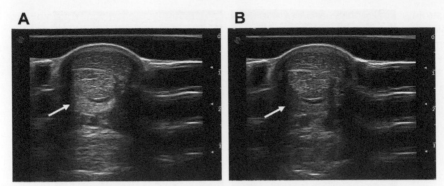

Fig. 6. Transverse images of the mid-metacarpus (lateral is to the left of the images). (*A*) Ultrasound beam is perpendicular to the fibers of the flexor tendons and inferior check ligament (*arrow*), which have a normal echogenicity. (*B*) The ultrasound beam is no longer perpendicular to the fibers of the deep digital flexor tendon and inferior check ligament (*arrow*), creating an artifactual hypoechogenicity throughout these structures called an off-incidence artifact. This artifact can be purposefully used in some patients to better delineate the margins of the flexor tendons and help better visualize healed core lesions.

mechanical articulated arms to determine position.[6] Extended field-of-view imaging (**Fig. 7**) produces a composite still-frame image of multiple successive frames recorded by the machine as the probe moves over a long distance and possibly curved surfaces, without the use of any positioning devices. In addition, a large lesion or structure can now be measured on a single image. In one study using an ultrasound phantom, linear measurements obtained with the extended field-of-view images were all within 5% of the known values.[6] One disadvantage of the technology is that obtaining a diagnostic extended field-of-view image takes practice, as it requires a very steady movement of the probe with a constant speed. Such a maneuver can be especially difficult if the patient is moving or the lesion/structure of interest covers a large area.

One of the main advantages of ultrasonography over other imaging modalities is the ability to view patient anatomy in real time. The dynamic ultrasonographic examination is primarily used for determining the presence of adhesion formation and evaluation of

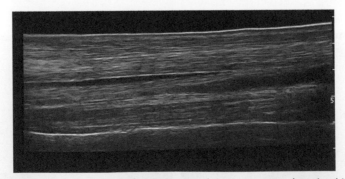

Fig. 7. Longitudinal extended field-of-view image of the metacarpus (proximal is to the left of the image). Instead of only visualizing 4 to 5 cm of the metacarpal tendons/ligaments, almost the entire length of the metacarpus can be recorded in one image; this is especially helpful in documenting the full extent of a lesion.

gastrointestinal motility, and to guide needle placement for sample collection or intra-lesional treatments. Video clips or cine loops of varying duration can be recorded to demonstrate a region of interest, and are helpful when reviewing the examination at a later time. These clips are especially useful for comparing repeated examinations of the same structure or lesion, as they provide a more real-time documentation of the examination. The disadvantage of video clips is the amount of space needed to save and store the large data files.

As the tissues evaluated with ultrasonography are 3-dimensional (3D), it seems reasonable to evaluate and depict these structures in a 3D image. Ultrasonographic images can now be created and displayed in 3D, using volume imaging software. A volume of data can be acquired by 3 different methods: freehand (with or without an external tracking device), a mechanically swept transducer, or a 2-dimensional (2D) transducer than can acquire 3D data.[7] The data obtained are reconstructed and displayed as either multiplanar (3 orthogonal slices) or volume-rendered images on the ultrasonogram. The images are useful when evaluating more complex anatomy or irregularly shaped structures or lesions. Linear and volume measurements of the structure of interest can also be obtained with 3D postprocessing, which has been shown to be more accurate than 2D linear measurements and helpful when trying to decide if a structure is truly enlarged.[5,7–9] Four-dimensional (adding time to 3D) imaging can be obtained by displaying these images as real-time presentations. This technology is quite popular in human obstetrics, cardiology, and gynecology,[10] yet currently has limited availability in veterinary medicine. These images are very helpful for teaching students, educating owners, and in recheck examinations; however, whether this technology will improve the diagnostic yield of the modality and impact management of equine clinical cases is yet to be determined.

During a sonographic examination, the size, homogeneity, echogenicity and, in some cases, dynamic movement of tissues can be evaluated. Although not commonly used in veterinary applications, ultrasonography can also measure the mechanical properties of tissues, such as elasticity. As a tissue is compressed (ie, by a transducer), the acoustic properties of the tissues change as they are strained or loaded. This change can be measured by tracking the distortion of the tissues and, as expected, soft tissues are more compressible than hard tissues. A color map is superimposed on the gray-scale image to depict different tissue stiffnesses[8] (yellow to red for softer tissues and green to blue for harder tissues) (**Fig. 8**). In human musculoskeletal imaging, this technology has been used to help identify areas of abnormality within tendons that may be isoechoic to normal tissue.[8] The research performed so far in equine tendons is limited,[11] and the clinical use of elastography in the evaluation of tendon/ligament healing is unknown at this time.

Ultrasound-guided interventional procedures, such as biopsies, fine-needle aspi-rates, and intralesional injections, have been performed for years. However, the diffi-culty with these procedures, primarily for inexperienced sonographers, is often correctly aligning the needle and visualizing it on the screen. For the needle trajectory to be completely visible, the needle has to be in the precise plane of the ultrasound beam, which varies but is typically only about 1 mm in width. Multiple needle-tracking devices have been tried to help guide the sonographer, many of which are currently used in human medicine.[12] Needle guides can be attached to the transducer to help maintain alignment of the needle with the ultrasound beam; however, in the authors' experience these devices can be bulky and prevent quick removal of the transducer if the patient suddenly moves. Recently, electromagnetic tracking systems have been developed and tested for use in freehand interventional procedures.[13,14] Using one sensor in the needle tip and another sensor either on or built into the

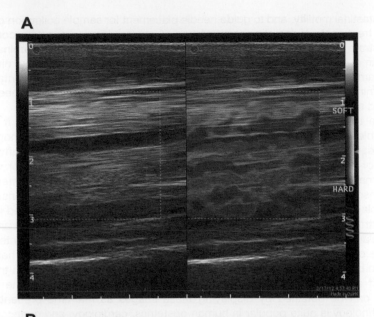

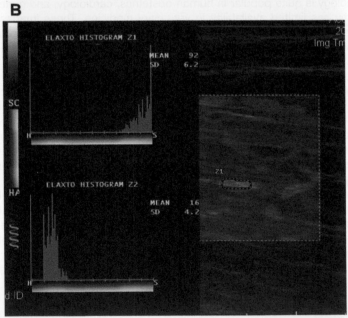

Fig. 8. Longitudinal elastography images of the mid-metacarpus (proximal is to the left of the images). (*A*) Color map of varying tissue stiffnesses of the palmar metacarpal structures. Yellow, orange, and red are for softer tissues while green to blue is for stiffer tissues. (*B*) Regions of interest can be drawn within certain anatomic structures, and a histogram of the tissue's elasticity is generated.

transducer, the needle track can be identified on the screen at all times during the procedure.[15] This technology is especially useful for those who do not perform these procedures on a regular basis or for practitioners performing intralesional therapies, to ensure the injection goes into the appropriate location. However, the use of electromagnetic technology in veterinary medicine is currently limited.

Fusion imaging is a new development in ultrasound technology and is not yet widely available. Image fusion allows combination of cross-sectional imaging data, such as from a CT or MRI examination, into the live ultrasonographic examination. This software uses navigator technology and anatomic landmarks, such as bony structures, to correctly combine the different modalities, showing the real-time ultrasonographic examination on one side of the screen with the corresponding MRI/CT slice on the other side. An electromagnetic tracking system is mounted on the ultrasound probe and CT/MRI data are altered as the transmitter detects probe movement.[8] This technique may be helpful for correlating lesions on prior MRI examinations with follow-up ultrasonographic examinations or to guide intralesional therapy.

Although these advancements in ultrasound equipment and software make scanning easier by improving the image and decreasing artifacts, the basic principles still need to be applied. Learning how to optimize the image, manipulate the transducer, and interpret the examination is a skill that takes time and practice to master. Not all ultrasound machines are created equal, so understanding the limitations and available software applications of the machine currently used in each individual equine practice is very important. Images on different machines with similar frequency transducers can look markedly different with baseline machine settings. With the help of a company representative, baseline settings such as gray scale, dynamic range, and spatial compounding, among others, can be adjusted to optimize the image settings to the sonographer's preferences. The fundamentals of ultrasound scanning can be acquired through the increasing number of continuing education courses available and then followed by practice on one's own machine to develop the necessary skills.

In summary, ultrasonography is a very popular and attractive imaging modality for use in equine practice, owing to its relatively low cost, ease of use, lack of ionizing radiation, and ability to be performed in the standing patient. The advancements in ultrasound technology, including better image resolution, compound imaging, harmonic imaging, extended-field-of-view, cine loops, 3D imaging, elastography, and fusion imaging are increasing the ability of ultrasonography to detect abnormalities, assess healing, and document lesions. However, as the resolution of ultrasonography improves and images become clearer, care must be taken to understand the variations from normal, and not to overinterpret the information being presented on the screen.

REFERENCES

1. Werpy N. Advancements in ultrasound. In: Proceedings North American Veterinary Conference. Orlando (FL): Eastern States Veterinary Association; 2008. p. 273–4.
2. Denoix JM, Farres D. Ultrasonographic imaging of the proximal third interosseous muscle in the pelvic limb using a plantaromedial approach. J Equine Vet Sci 1995;15:346–50.
3. Kremkau FW. Sonography: principles and instruments. St Louis (MO): Elsevier; 2011. p. 69–123.
4. Entrekin RR, Porter BA, Sillesen HH, et al. Real time spatial compound imaging: application to breast, vascular, and musculoskeletal ultrasound. Semin Ultrasound CT MR 2001;22(1):50–64.

5. Diaz JF, Guillermo AR, Matas RB, et al. New technologies applied to ultrasound diagnosis of sports injuries. Adv Ther 2008;25(12):1315–30.
6. Weng L, Tirumalai AP, Lowery CM, et al. US extended-field-of-view imaging technology. Radiology 1997;203:877–80.
7. Prager RW, Ijaz UA, Gee AH, et al. Three-dimensional ultrasound imaging. In: Proceedings of the Institution of Mechanical Engineers, Part H. Journal of Engineering in Medicine 2010; 224:193–223.
8. Klauser AS, Peetrons P. Developments in musculoskeletal ultrasound and clinical applications. Skeletal Radiol 2010;39:1061–71.
9. Riccabona M, Nelson TR, Pretorius DH. Three dimensional ultrasound: accuracy of distance and volume measurements. Ultrasound Obstet Gynecol 1996;7: 429–34.
10. Nelson TR. Three-dimensional ultrasound imaging. Proceedings Ultrasonic Industry Association (UIA) Annual Meeting. San Diego (CA): Institute of Electrical and Electronic Engineers; 2006. p. 1–5.
11. Crevier-Denoix N, Ravary-Plumioën B, Evrard D, et al. Reproducibility of a non-invasive ultrasonic technique of tendon force measurement, determined in vitro in equine superficial digital flexor tendons. J Biomech 2009;42:2210–3.
12. Souzdalnitski D, Lerman I, Halaszynski TM. How to improve needle visibility. In: Narouze SN, editor. Atlas of ultrasound-guided procedures in interventional pain management. New York: Springer; 2011. p. 35–75.
13. Hakime A, Deschamps F, De Carvalho E, et al. Electromagnetic-tracked biopsy under ultrasound guidance: preliminary results [published online ahead of print September 27 2011]. Cardiovasc Intervent Radiol 2011. Available at: http://www.springerlink.com/content/. Accessed May 7, 2012.
14. Levy EB, Tang J, Lindisch D, et al. Implementation of an electromagnetic tracking system for accurate intrahepatic puncture needle guidance; accuracy results in an in vitro model. Acad Radiol 2007;14(3):344–53.
15. Pollard BA. Ultrasound guidance for vascular access and regional anesthesia. Toronto: Library and Archives Canada; 2011. p. 23–27.

Imaging of the Equine Proximal Suspensory Ligament

Natasha M. Werpy, DVM, DACVR[a],*, Jean-Marie Denoix, DVM, PhD[b]

KEYWORDS

- Suspensory ligament • Metacarpals • Imaging modalities • Anisotropy

KEY POINTS

- A thorough knowledge of anatomy is required to be proficient at ultrasonographic examination of the proximal suspensory ligament.
- All modalities can contribute valuable information about osseous lesions at the attachment of the suspensory ligament on the third metacarpal and metatarsal bones.
- Multiple approaches are necessary to perform a complete ultrasound examination of the proximal suspensory ligament.
- Magnetic resonance imaging (MRI) will be required to diagnose certain types of suspensory ligament injury.

INTRODUCTION

Suspensory ligament (SL) injury is an important source of lameness in performance horses.[1,2] Injury to the SL not only affects the ligament; the third metacarpal or metatarsal bone may also be affected.[3,4] Multiple modalities are available to aid in the diagnosis of SL injury.[5] All modalities can make a contribution to the diagnosis and characterization of SL injury. Because of the combination of soft-tissue and osseous injuries that can occur, multiple modalities are often required to fully characterize SL injury. The purpose of this article is to describe the advantages each imaging modality in the diagnosis of SL injury, to describe a method for examination of the SL using ultrasound (US), and to provide a better understanding of why advanced imaging will be required for a diagnosis in certain cases.

ANATOMY OF THE SL

The anatomy of the SL is complicated. To properly use imaging for a diagnosis, it is imperative to understand the anatomy of the structure or region of interest. The

[a] Diagnostic Imaging, University of Florida, College of Veterinary Medicine, Gainesville, Florida, USA; [b] Anatomy and Lameness Diagnosis in Horses, CIRALE-Hippolia - 14430 Goustranville, France INRA, USC BPLC 957 - Université Paris-Est, Ecole Nationale Vétérinaire d'Alfort - 94704 Maisons-Alfort, France
* Corresponding author. Small Animal Clinical Sciences University of Florida College of Veterinary Medicine Gainesville, FL 32656, USA.
E-mail address: equinedxim@yahoo.com

Vet Clin Equine 28 (2012) 507–525
http://dx.doi.org/10.1016/j.cveq.2012.08.005
0749-0739/12/$ – see front matter

more complicated the anatomy, the greater knowledge required to make a correct diagnosis. It is well established that there are regions of fat and muscle in the SL.[6] These regions affect its appearance, particularly on US and advanced imaging. Although both the front and hind SLs have areas of fat and muscle, there are important anatomic differences when comparing them.[7]

Anatomy of the Forelimb SL

The SL in the forelimbs begins as a thin layer of fibers originating from the proximal palmar aspect of the third carpal and metacarpal bones. Its bilobed appearance becomes readily apparent at the level of the attachment on the third metacarpal bone. Typically the medial lobe is thinner and wider than the lateral lobe (**Fig. 1**). However, this can vary among horses and even when comparing the right and left forelimbs of a horse. The palmar margin of the third metacarpal bone has often a focal sagittal osseous crest at the attachment of the SL, and this should not be confused with abnormal osseous proliferation. At the level where the SL is bilobed, focal regions of fat and muscle are contained within each lobe to varying degrees. When comparing the medial and lateral lobes in a forelimb, both the amount and distribution are variable. Furthermore, this appearance can be similar or quite asymmetric when comparing the opposite limb. Although the regions of fat and muscle are most often contained within the lobes, they can dissect through the SL fibers to the periphery of the ligament. Approximately 5 to 6 cm distal to the carpometacarpal joint the medial and lateral lobes of the SL join together to form an oval ligament (Vet Radiol Ultrasound, in review). This oval shape continues distally to the level of the bifurcation. Once the lobes join together the fat and muscle remain well defined but become more dispersed throughout the ligament, typically in a zig zag pattern with less muscle at this level. The muscle does not continue into the SL branches.

In addition to understanding the anatomy of the ligament, it is important to recognize its relationship to adjacent anatomic structures. Although the forelimb SL is relatively centered on the palmar aspect of the third metacarpal bone, there are anatomic characteristics that affect what part of the SL is visible when imaging with US from the palmar margin of the limb. Although the superficial digital flexor

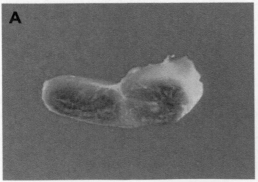 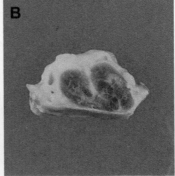

Fig. 1. Gross anatomic sections demonstrating the normal anatomy of the front and hind suspensory ligaments. Both sections were obtained immediately distal to the osseous attachment. The front suspensory ligament (A) has the typical appearance of a thin but wide medial lobe, and a thicker but narrower lateral lobe. The hind suspensory ligament (B) is heart shaped with a larger dorsal to plantar thickness. The muscle can be identified as pink tissue interspersed with regions of white fat surrounded by ligament fibers. Medial is to the left on both images.

tendon (SDFT) is mildly thicker medially, the deep digital flexor tendon (DDFT) and the inferior check ligament, or accessory ligament of the deep digital flexor tendon (AL-DDFT), are thicker laterally. The anatomic characteristics of the palmar soft tissues at the level of the third metacarpal bone affect the contact surface (contact area for the probe) on the palmar aspect of the limb. In addition, the medial lobe is wider (longer in the medial to lateral direction) when compared with the lateral lobe. The bulk of palmar metacarpal tissues lateral of midline in conjunction with a narrower lateral lobe results in greater visualization of the lateral lobe from the palmar aspect of the limb.

Anatomy of the Forelimb Vasculature and Nerves

The blood supply of the SL comes from the lateral (third) and medial (second) palmar metacarpal arteries descending at the palmar aspect of the third metacarpal bone. These arteries originate from the radial artery medially and the ulnar collateral artery laterally. Close to the carpometacarpal joint these arteries are connected by a deep palmar arch that transversely crosses the palmar aspect of the proximal suspensory ligament (PSL) providing the metacarpal arteries. A satellite venous deep palmar arch between the lateral and medial palmar metacarpal veins is seen at the palmar and dorsal aspects of the PSL. The venous drainage is made through the collateral ulnar vein laterally and the cephalic vein medially.

The SL is innervated by a deep ramus originating from the palmar ramus of the ulnar nerve at the level of the distal row of the carpus. These rami have integrated nerve fibers coming from an anastomosis arising from the median nerve.

The palmar metacarpal arteries and veins are quite prominent at the proximal aspect of the third metacarpal bone. At the level of the carpometacarpal joint they are located palmar medial and palmar lateral to the SL. These vessels converge and track dorsal and palmar to the ligament, as well as palmar medial and palmar lateral throughout the length of the third metacarpal bone.

Anatomy of the Hindlimb SL

The SL in the hind limb begins as a triangular shape at the proximal aspect of the third metatarsal bone. The triangle is thinner medially than it is laterally. The SL is closer to the fourth metatarsal bone, with a larger amount of connective tissue separating it from the second metatarsal bone. The anatomic relationship between the hind SL and the fourth metatarsal bone is important when considering US examination of this structure. As the ligament continues distally it becomes heart shaped to round and then oval, until it reaches the level of the bifurcation. Throughout the transitions in shape of the SL, the apex of the triangle and the heart shape, which is the plantar margin of the ligament, is directed plantar lateral. Therefore, the majority of the SL is lateral of midline and adjacent to the axial margin of the fourth metatarsal bone. The relationship becomes less important distally as the size of the fourth metatarsal bone decreases relative to the SL. In contrast to the SL in the forelimb, the hind SL typically has a prominent area of central fibers as well as peripheral fibers, and is not bilobed (see **Fig. 1**). The fat and muscle distribution is more similarly positioned when comparing medial and lateral aspects of the ligament, in contrast to the variable appearance in the forelimb. However, random areas of fat and muscle can still dissect through the ligament to the peripheral margin, and asymmetry between limbs still exists. These regions should not be mistaken for injury. Similar to the SL in the forelimb, regions of fat and muscle converge into a zig zag pattern as the ligament takes on an oval shape.

Anatomy of the Hindlimb Vasculature and Nerves

The blood supply of the hind SL comes from the medial (second) and lateral (third) plantar metatarsal arteries. The blood flow mainly comes from the perforating tarsal artery originating at the dorsolateral aspect of the hock from the dorsal pedal artery and passing in the tarsal canal. The perforating tarsal artery supplies the plantar metatarsal arch receiving the small plantar arteries and providing the second and third plantar metatarsal arteries. The venous drainage is mainly achieved by a large second plantar metatarsal vein continuing in the tarsal canal as a perforating tarsal vein joining the cranial tibial veins through the dorsal pedal veins.

Innervation of the hind SL is provided by the deep ramus of the lateral plantar nerve coming from the tibial nerve. This ramus originates at the level of the proximal intertarsal joint and provides several fasciculi for the SL and distal plantar ligament.

Summary points

- The PSL in the forelimb is bilobed, and the lobes fuse together to form an oval ligament until the level of the bifurcation.

- The most common appearance of the PSL in the forelimb is a wide, thin medial lobe and a narrow, thick lateral lobe. Although it is less common, the PSL in the forelimb can have lobes that are symmetric in size.

- The fat and muscle can vary in distribution between limbs and horses in the fore and hind limbs, and can dissect through the SL fibers in normal horses.

- The PSL in the hind limb is triangular and then often becomes heart shaped before becoming oval. The ligament remains oval until the level of the bifurcation.

RADIOGRAPHY

Horizontal dorsopalmar/plantar, lateromedial, and oblique radiographic projections can all provide information about the proximal metacarpal/tarsal region relative to SL injury.[4,8] The proximal metacarpal/tarsal region should be fully evaluated for any osseous abnormalities. The trabecular bone pattern in the proximal aspect of the third metacarpal/tarsal bone is of particular interest. The second and fourth metacarpal/tarsal bones and their relationship to the third metacarpal/tarsal bone should also be assessed. Any osseous proliferation on the second and fourth metacarpal/tarsal bones should be noted, as further investigation will be required to determine its relationship, if any, to the margins of the SL. Thickening of the palmar/plantar cortex of the third metacarpal/tarsal bones is best seen on lateromedial projections, whereas abnormalities in the trabecular bone pattern are best identified on dorsopalmar/plantar views.

Regions of sclerosis, radiolucency, and/or avulsion fracture at the attachment of the SL on the third metacarpal/tarsal bone can be diagnosed radiographically. Radiographs can also identify abnormalities that may appear as SL injury based on clinical presentation and blocking, such as incomplete palmar metacarpal fractures. Therefore, complete and detailed evaluation of all anatomy on radiographs is important. The distal carpus and tarsus should also be evaluated, as these regions can block

---

Summary points

- Radiographs can reveal osseous abnormalities associated with the SL attachment on the third metacarpal or metatarsal bone.

- A normal radiograph study does not rule out SL disease or associated osseous injury.

similarly to the proximal metacarpal/tarsal region. A lack of osseous abnormalities on radiographs does not rule out SL injury, and nuclear scintigraphy can demonstrate osseous injury that may not be radiographically visible.

SCINTIGRAPHY

Soft-tissue and bone phase images can be used to evaluate the proximal metacarpal/tarsal regions. Focal scintigraphic uptake in the proximal metacarpal/tarsal region on bone phase images can be seen for many different types of injuries including bone resorption, sclerosis, palmar metacarpal cortical fracture, and fluid deposition (**Fig. 2**). Nuclear scintigraphy can also provide information about other injuries, such as carpal or tarsal bone diseases, which can mimic SL injury in clinical presentation and at the same time provide evidence of any additional osseous issues with increased bone turnover. Additional imaging is required to characterize the increased radiopharmaceutical uptake (IRU). Bone fluid or edema diagnosed with magnetic resonance imaging (MRI) can often be monitored with subsequent nuclear scintigraphy examinations.

False-negative information, such as no IRU on soft-tissue phase images, can be seen in horses with PSL disease established with nerve blocks and US.

Summary points

- Nuclear scintigraphy examination can demonstrate areas of increased bone turnover associated with the SL attachment.

- Further imaging is required to determine the cause of IRU.

- Radiographs and computed tomography (CT) can demonstrate the presence of sclerosis, and enthesophyte formation or resorption. US can be used to identify change in peripheral bone margin. However, MRI is required to determine if there is fluid in the bone.

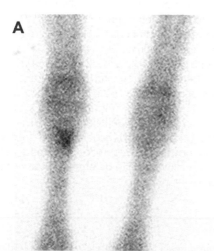
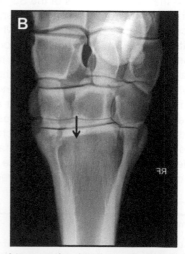

Fig. 2. Skeletal scintigraphy examination with focal increased radiopharmaceutical uptake (IRU) in the right proximal metacarpal region (*A*), and the corresponding dorsopalmar radiograph (*B*). The IRU in the third metacarpal bone corresponds to a region of radiolucency (*black arrow*) indicating bone loss or resorption bordered by sclerosis at the attachment of the medial lobe of the suspensory ligament.

ULTRASONOGRAPHY

US is an extremely useful tool for the diagnosis of SL injury. However, as described in this section, diagnosis of SL injury often requires the clinician to go above and beyond the techniques that can provide a diagnosis for the flexor tendons. This section explains why altering the direction of the ultrasound beam is necessary to visualize the SL anatomy and is required to identify pathologic change. It covers additional techniques that should be used in conjunction with the standard technique of SL US to provide a comprehensive examination. Do not be put off by the physics paragraph; it is really straightforward, and necessary to properly scan the SL sonographically.

Anisotropy: One of the US Physics Principles that Really Matters!

The complicated anatomy of the SL requires additional US techniques to be used for complete visualization of the ligament and to correctly identify its anatomy. One of the challenges of SL US is that the regions of fat and muscle create variations in the ligament echogenicity. This echo pattern makes it difficult to determine if these variations in echogenicity are the result of injury or the normal SL anatomy. A technique that can be used to correctly identify regions of SL fibers versus areas of fat and muscle is called off-angle or oblique-incidence imaging. The basis for this technique is the US physics principle of anisotropy. This principle is demonstrated every time the angle of the ultrasound probe is adjusted proximally or distally to create maximum echogenicity when examining the palmar metacarpal flexor tendons in the transverse plane. When the ultrasound beam is truly perpendicular to the longitudinal axis of linear fibers within a normal tendon, maximum echogenicity is created. When the ultrasound beam is not perpendicular to a normal tendon, decreased echogenicity can be created in that structure. In contrast to normal tendon or ligament fibers, the echogenicity of fat and, to a lesser degree, muscle is not dependent on the angle of the ultrasound beam. The difference between the echogenicity of SL fibers and that of the regions of fat and muscle becomes very apparent when the ultrasound beam is not perpendicular to the longitudinal axis of the SL fibers. This change in the position of the probe can be used to identify regions of fibers versus regions of fat and muscle.

Normal SL fibers will be echogenic when the ultrasound beam is perpendicular to the longitudinal axis of the fibers and will become hypoechogenic when the beam is no longer perpendicular to the fibers. By contrast, regions of fat and, to a lesser degree, muscle will remain echogenic regardless of beam angle. Therefore, comparing the appearance of the SL with the beam both perpendicular and not perpendicular to the ligament allows identification of fibers versus regions of fat and muscle (Vet Radiol Ultrasound, in review). Therefore, regions of mottling or decreased echogenicity identified in the SL with US can then be further investigated using changes in beam angle to determine if the source of the these regions is ligament fibers or fat and muscle. This technique provides a method for determining the actual tissue source, which allows one to determine whether this is part of a normal pattern of the SL or a region of injury.

Summary points

- SL fibers will be echogenic when the ultrasound beam is perpendicular to the longitudinal axis of the ligament fibers and will markedly decrease in echogenicity when the ultrasound beam is not perpendicular.

- Fat and muscle fibers demonstrate mild changes in echogenicity with changes in beam angle, and relative to SL fibers, fat and muscle will remain echogenic regardless of beam angle.

Similar to the areas of fat and muscle, the echogenicity of the connective tissue surrounding the SL is not beam angle dependent (remains echogenic regardless of beam angle). Placing the ultrasound beam slightly oblique to the SL allows differentiation of the ligament margins from the surrounding echogenic connective tissue.

Standard Approach in the Forelimb

Longitudinal and transverse images of the SL should be acquired from the palmar aspect of the limb. A linear probe is used for examination of the metacarpal region. The frequency, focal zones, depth, and gain should be adjusted to maximize image quality at the level of the SL. Although all structures at this level should be assessed during the US examination, the depth should be set such that the hyperechoic line representing the palmar margin of the third metacarpal bone is clearly visible. Comparison with the opposite limb is imperative in all cases. Even in cases with obvious SL injury, additional findings become apparent when compared with the opposite leg. A measurement system (zones or centimeters distal to the accessory carpal bone) should be consistently used. The palmar approach with a linear probe creates a rectangular appearance to the SL.[9] As previously discussed in the anatomy section, the width of the PSL is greater than the AL-DDFT and the flexor tendons. Therefore, the contact area of the ultrasound probe with the palmar margin of the leg creates this rectangular appearance. The ultrasound beam can only penetrate the SL at the same width as the contact area when a linear probe is used. It is important to recognize that the SL extends beyond these margins, and additional techniques are required to fully image the ligament (**Fig. 3**). Two additional techniques are discussed in the following sections. However, using the standard approach the probe can be angled toward the second and fourth metacarpal bones while positioned on the palmar aspect of the limb to obtain images of the periphery of the SL.

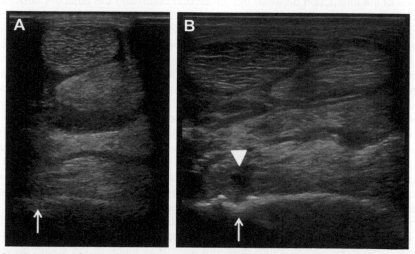

Fig. 3. US images of the case shown in **Fig. 2** (medial is to the left). Images were obtained using the standard technique (*A*) with the limb weight bearing, and using the non–weight-bearing technique with the limb flexed (*B*). Both images were obtained with beam angle perpendicular to the longitudinal axis of the fibers. The lesion is not readily apparent using the standard technique. Focal bone irregularity can be identified at the edge of the image (*arrow* in *A*). By contrast, focal bone resorption (*arrow*) and ligament injury (*arrowhead*) are well identified with the flexed limb (*B*).

The SL has a mottled appearance as a result of the regions of fat and muscle within the ligament. This mottled appearance will create regions of decreased echogenicity in the ligament on transverse images and regions with nonlinear fibers when evaluating the ligament longitudinally. With the increase in image resolution and detection of tissue planes now available with portable US machines, the interfaces between fibers and regions of fat and muscle are more apparent. Given the differences in imaging properties, converting from an analog to digital US machine requires an adjustment in evaluation and interpretation of the SL.

The entire SL body should be evaluated in transverse and longitudinal planes with images obtained at regular measurement intervals. The size, shape, margins, and echogenicity should be evaluated.

Summary points

- The frequency, focal zones, depth, and gain should be adjusted to maximize image quality at the level of the SL.

- It is important to recognize that the peripheral margins of the ligament are not visualized using the standard approach.

- Size, shape, margins, and echogenicity of the SL should be evaluated in longitudinal and transverse planes with a consistent measurement method so that recheck examinations can be performed appropriately.

Understanding the Effect of Edge Artifacts and Vasculature on the SL when Using the Standard Approach

The importance of understanding the effect of edge artifacts and through-transmission on the appearance of the SL when using the standard approach cannot be underestimated. Both artifacts cause alterations in the echogenicity of the SL as a result of the interaction between the ultrasound beam and the adjacent structures.

Edge artifact occurs when the sound beam hits a curved surface and is deflected away from the ultrasound probe. The deflected sound beam then never returns back to the ultrasound probe; consequently the machine has no information about this area and it appears as a black line on the image. Using a palmar metacarpal vessel as an example, the sound wave leaves the ultrasound probe and travels toward the vessel. When it encounters the palmar and dorsal margins of the vessel it is reflected back to the US machine, creating an anechoic circular structure bordered palmar dorsally by white lines. However, the angle of the medial and lateral vessel margins causes the sound wave to be deflected away from the ultrasound probe. The medial and lateral vessel walls do not have the same double echogenic lines associated with the dorsal and palmar walls. In addition, extending from the medial and lateral vessels walls are hypoechoic lines extending through the tissues deep to the vessel. This situation can occur with any curved structure when the sound beam encounters the interface at an oblique angle, such as the SDFT in the metacarpus or the DDFT in the metatarsus.

Through-transmission, also called distal acoustic enhancement, causes an artifactual increase in echogenicity in tissue that is deep to a fluid-filled structure, such as a vessel. The fluid-filled structure does not absorb as much of the sound beam as the adjacent tissue at the same level. As the sound beam continues along its path, the tissue deep to the fluid-filled structure encounters a stronger or less attenuated ultrasound beam. A stronger beam returns to the ultrasound probe and is interpreted by the machine as brighter or more echogenic tissue. Any tissue deep to a vessel or other fluid-filled structure will appear brighter than the adjacent tissue that is at the same depth.

   Edge artifact and through-transmission occur simultaneously as the sound beam encounters a vessel. When trying to decipher this pattern it is easier to identify the structures that could be affecting the echogenicity of the SL before evaluating the ligament itself. Using the metacarpal region as an example, identify the edge artifacts resulting from any soft-tissue structures, such as the SDFT, and follow it dorsally to identify where it crosses the SL (**Fig. 4**). Identify the vessels palmar to the SL, and follow the edge artifacts from the margins dorsally and determine where they cross the SL. Next, look at the width and depth of the vessels palmar to the SL and evaluate the corresponding echo pattern in the SL. The further away the vessel is located, the less effect it will have on the echogenicity of the SL. Follow the vessels dorsally to the SL, with an expectation of increased echogenicity in the SL fibers that are dorsal to vessels. Using the same thought process, the regions of the SL not affected by through-transmission (no adjacent vessels) should be relatively less echogenic when compared with the regions affected by through-transmission. Once this

---

Summary points

- A visual survey of the anatomy should be performed as a first step in the US examination. Any structures that may affect the echogenicity of the SL can then be identified.

- Based on the artifacts (edge artifact or through transmission), an expected pattern of variations in echogenicity of the SL will be observed. The echogenicity of the SL is interpreted in light of this expected pattern.

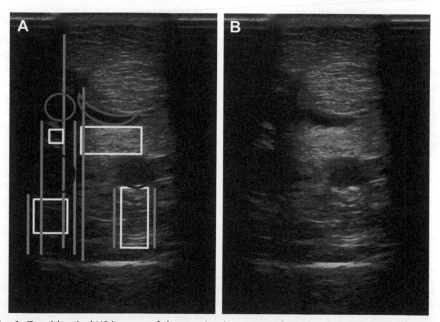

Fig. 4. Two identical US images of the proximal metacarpal region. Image *A* depicts areas of through transmission (*yellow boxes*) caused by vessels (*red and blue circles* = artery and veins) and the carpal canal (*green crescent*). The edge artifacts (*orange lines*) are the result of vessel and flexor tendon margins. Image *A* can then be compared with image *B* to fully appreciate the echogenicity pattern resulting from these artifacts. These artifacts should be identified and their potential effects on the appearance of the suspensory ligament determined before evaluating the ligament for abnormalities.

evaluation is completed, the SL ligament can be evaluated with an expected echo pattern based on surrounding structures. Abnormalities in the ligament will alter this expected echo pattern.

Complements to the Standard Approach in the Forelimb: Medial and Lateral Approach and Use of a Stand-Off Pad

Once the standard approach is completed from the palmar aspect of the limb, the ultrasound probe is then moved to either the medial or lateral aspect of the limb. The ultrasound probe is placed as proximally as is possible to allow visualization of the peripheral surface of the SL that is not obscured by the second or fourth metacarpal bones. This approach will allow visualization of the curved peripheral ligament margin, which is not visible from the palmar aspect of the limb (**Fig. 5**). This technique should be part of the standard examination, but is especially important when peripheral swelling is present that is not associated with the AL-DDFT or other palmar metacarpal structures. This approach also allows visualization of periligamentous tissue proliferation and evaluation of the relationship between the SL and the palmar metacarpal fascia, a thin layer of fibrous connective tissue that extends from the palmar margin of the second and fourth metacarpal bones around the palmar soft tissues. Periligamentous tissue proliferation is often more prominent along the medial and lateral peripheral margins of the ligament, when compared with the palmar margin, and again cannot be accurately evaluated from the palmar aspect of the limb. The medial and lateral margins of the SL should be examined separately. This examination often requires the use of a stand-off pad. However, it may not be necessary when swelling in the region of the SL is present. A stand-off pad can be used with the standard approach from the palmar aspect of the limb, and will mildly increase the contact surface between the probe and the skin surface. Very thin stand-off pads are now available, which minimally affect or attenuate the sound beam and can be used with minimal consequence to the US image quality. A stand-off pad can be used with any of these techniques providing it improves visualization of the ligament, and that this improvement is not offset by a decrease in detail or an increase in artifact resulting from its use. The medial and lateral approach and use of stand off pad can be applied in the hind limb.

Summary points

- Placing the probe on the medial and lateral aspects of the limb is the best method for imaging SL edge lesions, associated periligamentous tissue proliferation, and the palmar metacarpal fascia in this region.

- A stand-off pad can be used to augment any technique when improved visualization of the SL is achieved.

Non–Weight-Bearing Technique

In addition to the standard approach, the SL should be examined with the limb mildly flexed at the carpus (**Fig. 6**). The minimal amount of carpal flexion that can be maintained with the limb in a steady position will allow the best visualization of the SL origin. If the horse is resistant in maintaining this position, the carpus can be maintained at a more flexed position once the proximal 4 cm of the SL body has been examined. The increased carpal flexion will still allow examination of the remaining SL body. Examining the SL with the carpus flexed allows improved visualization of the SL when compared with the standard approach (Vet Radiol Ultrasound, in review) (see **Fig. 3**). Flexion of the carpus results in relaxation of the palmar soft tissues. The flexor

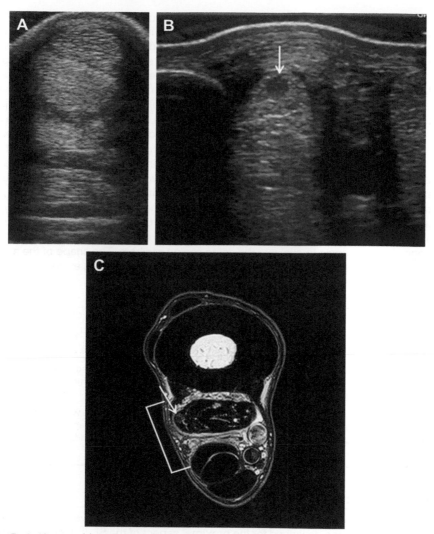

Fig. 5. A 12-year-old Hanoverian gelding jumper presented with grade 1 lameness, focal lateral swelling of the proximal metacarpal region, and pain on palpation of the SL. US images obtained using the standard (*A*) and the lateral approach (*B*; white box on *C* shows position of the ultrasound probe), and corresponding MR image (*C*). Focal injury (*white arrows*) to the lateral aspect of the SL was not diagnosed with standard approach, and was better visualized with lateral approach than with examination performed on the flexed limb. The injury to the SL fibers was confirmed on an MR study, and no additional injuries to the ligament were identified.

tendons can then be manipulated, which will increase the contact area for the ultrasound probe. The entire SL is now visible in one image, in contrast to the standard technique. The manipulation of the flexor tendons decreases the depth between the ultrasound probe and the SL. The decrease in depth increases image detail by allowing the use of a higher frequency. In addition to manipulation of the flexor tendons, the vasculature can be more easily manipulated. Although the anastomosis of the deep palmar arch of the palmar metacarpal arteries still creates artifact overlying the SL, the extensive edge artifact and through-transmission artifacts are substantially decreased with this technique (Vet Radiol Ultrasound, in review). This method allows visualization of the relationship between the second and fourth metacarpal bones and the SL. Axial margin proliferation on the margins of the second and fourth metacarpal bones along with syndesmoses can be more easily identified. In addition, increased detail achieved with this method allows careful assessment of potential contact areas between the axial metacarpal bone (second and fourth) proliferation and the margins of the SL. It is important to note is that this method can falsely give the appearance of contact between axial metacarpal bone proliferation and the SL. The laxity of the flexor tendons and pressure of the ultrasound probe can push the SL into the margins of the metacarpal bones. This relationship may not exist in a similar fashion when the horse is in a weight-bearing position. Therefore, Contact between the axial margins of the metacarpal bones and the SL should be interpreted with caution in using this examination method. It is important to recognize that a change in the position of the ultrasound beam angle will result in evaluation of fibers proximal or distal to the original probe position. The ultrasound probe must be moved slightly proximal or distal with changes in beam angle to evaluate the same region of fibers. The shape of the adjacent bone margins can be used to ensure the same fibers are being evaluated during the changes in beam angle.

Summary points

- US of the SL with the limb flexed allows complete visualization of the SL, and varying the beam angle facilitates differentiation between SL fiber and regions of fat and muscle.

- This technique can be used to evaluate the relationship between the SL and axial margins of the second and fourth metacarpal bones. However, applied pressure during scanning can create a false appearance of contact between the SL and bone.

- To evaluate the same region of fibers at different ultrasound beam angles will require slight proximal or distal movement of the ultrasound probe. Comparing the shape of the bone margins can be used to ensure the on-beam and off-beam images are made at the same anatomic location.

Standard Approach in the Hind Limb

The standard technique for evaluation of the SL in the hind limb involves using a medial approach as has been described for the proximal aspect of the SL.[10] In certain cases, the mid to distal aspects of the SL body must be imaged from the plantar aspect of the limb, because at this location the medial aspect of the limb does not provide an adequate contact surface to allow visualization of the ligament even with a stand-off pad. As discussed in the anatomy section, the PSL is located adjacent to the fourth metatarsal bone. In addition, the axial margin of the fourth metatarsal bone, which is curved, wraps around the lateral margin of the SL and obscures it from view when imaging from the plantar aspect of the limb. By using the DDFT as a window and directing the ultrasound beam dorsal and lateral, the entire SL can be visualized. The hind SL changes shape more significantly than the front SL. In addition, subtle changes in shape as a result of ligament injury are often visible before fiber abnormalities are detected. Therefore, comparison with the opposite limb is imperative. In addition, the size and shape of the fourth metatarsal bone changes dramatically at the level of the PSL. The size and shape of the fourth metatarsal bone and its relationship to the third metatarsal bone can be used to ensure comparisons between the right and left hind limbs are being made at the same level (**Fig. 7**). As previously discussed in the standard approach

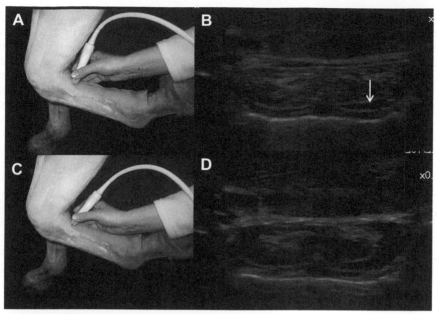

Fig. 6. Images depicting the position of limb and the probe for the non–weight-bearing US examination of the suspensory ligament, and corresponding US images. Image *A* shows probe perpendicular to the longitudinal axis of the SL creating echogenicity in ligament fibers (*B*). Image *C* shows probe not perpendicular to the ligament, and the resultant image has hypoechogenic fibers with echogenic fat and muscle (*D*). Note the slight decrease in echogenicity (*arrow*) in the dorsal aspect of the medial lobe (*B*). This appearance can be seen in normal suspensory ligaments.

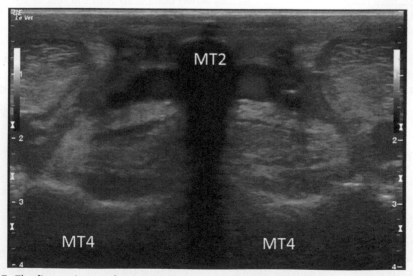

Fig. 7. The first author prefers to use mirror images to ensure the hind suspensory ligament is compared with the opposite limb at precisely the same level. The second author uses matched images (same orientation). The method that best clarifies the anatomy for each individual will aid in the detection of subtle abnormalities, such as the mild enlargement of the SL on the left.

of the forelimb, consistent measurement techniques and US machine settings that maximize image quality for SL imaging should be used. Evaluation of the SL margins for periligamentous tissue proliferation should be performed. The non–weight-bearing technique can be applied in the hind limb. It is often easier to see the fiber versus fat-muscle regions with the limb in a non–weight-bearing position (**Fig. 8**). Many injuries to the SL occur in the dorsal aspect of the ligament . Therefore, manipulating the flexor tendons with the limb in a non-weighte bearing position to allow the US beam to be oriented as dorsally as possible while still visualizing the entire ligament will aide in identifying abnormalities (**Fig. 9**).

Summary points

- The medial approach to the hind SL allows complete visualization of the ligament.
- The hind PSL changes shape dramatically as does the fourth metatarsal bone. Therefore, distinct anatomic landmarks, such as the shape of the fourth metatarsal bone, should be used when imaging the opposite limb for comparison.
- Imaging of the hind SL with the limb in a non–weight-bearing position facilitates the differentiation of SL fibers from regions of fat and muscle using variations in beam angle, as described for the forelimb.

Identifying Pathologic Change in the Forelimb and Hind Limb SL Using US

Abnormalities in the size, shape, margin, and echogenicity can all indicate abnormalities in the SL. Focal variations in the ligament echogenicity identified using the standard approach require further investigation with the limb in a non–weight-bearing position. Reexamining these regions with the limb in a non–weight-bearing position and varying ultrasound beam angles will establish if they are associated with SL fibers or regions of fat and muscle (**Fig. 3**). It is important to note is that the dorsal aspect of the SL may have decreased echogenicity when compared with the rest of the ligament, which may be the result of relaxation artifact. Further investigation of this appearance is warranted, but diffuse subtle decreased echogenicity in a ligament with a normal size and shape should be interpreted with caution. Regions of injury in the SL fibers will have decreased echogenicity regardless of beam angle (Vet Radiol Ultrasound, in review). These regions will appear as decreased echogenicity with the beam angle not perpendicular to the fibers. Their appearance will remain unchanged

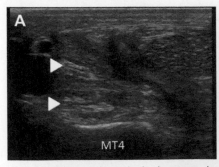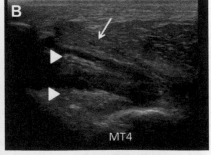

Fig. 8. US images made with the beam angle perpendicular (*A*) and oblique (*B*) to the hind SL with the limb mildly flexed. The regions of fat and muscle (*arrowheads*) remain echogenic regardless of beam angle. The tendon and ligament fibers become hypoechogenic with the ultrasound beam at an oblique angle. The periligamentous tissue proliferation (*arrow*) becomes more apparent adjacent to the hypoechogenic ligament fibers.

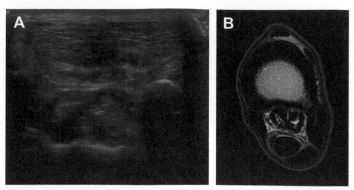

Fig. 9. Oblique incidence US image (*A*) made with the limb in a non-weight bearing position and corresponding MRI image (*B*) of a hind SL. The laxity of the flexor tendons with the limb in a non-weight bearing position permits manipulation of the soft tissue plantar to the SL. This manipulation allows a the US beam angle to be directed toward the plantar margin of the bone increasing visualization of the bone interface at the SL ligament attachment as well as more detailed imaging of the dorsal aspect of the ligament.

as the beam is moved perpendicular to the longitudinal axis of the SL and the surrounding normal fibers become echogenic. By contrast, scarring will be echogenic regardless of beam angle and can have associated ligament enlargement (Vet Radiol Ultrasound, in review). The echogenicity of mature fibrous tissue is independent of beam angle, creating its echogenic appearance despite changes in beam angle.

Injury to the SL often alters the fat and muscle distribution, and creates indistinct margins between regions of fibers and areas of fat and muscle. The regions of fat and muscle can become less evident with diffuse enlargement of the ligament and with focal regions of fiber injury and enlargement. Loss of the normal fat-muscle distribution in combination with abnormal fibers is often seen in conjunction with SL injury.

The margins of the SL should be closely examined. The examination is best done with the limb in a non–weight-bearing position and the ultrasound beam not perpendicular to the SL. Dorsal-margin fraying or tears and focal areas of enlargement along the dorsal border of the SL are best identified using this technique (Vet Radiol Ultrasound, in review) Abnormalities in the SL margin will be evident adjacent to echogenic connective tissue. It is important to recognize that some amount of edge artifact is present on the medial and lateral margins of the front SL, and on the dorsal and to a lesser degree the plantar margin in the hind SL, even using this technique. Therefore, small margin tears on the medial and lateral margins of the front SL will be best visualized using a medial or lateral approach, placing the ultrasound beam perpendicular to the affected margin (**Fig. 5**). This approach will also best identify periligamentous tissue proliferation and allow evaluation of the palmar metacarpal fascia on the medial and lateral aspect of the limbs.

Abnormalities in the palmar margin of the third metacarpal/tarsal bone will be recognized with the beam angle both perpendicular and not perpendicular to the osseous surface, as well as during evaluation in the longitudinal plane. However, the echogenicity of bone is beam angle dependent. The beam angle that best characterizes the appearance will depend on the lesion margins and configuration. The sagittal osseous crest on the palmar margin of the third metacarpal/tarsal bone can often appear prominent and may be mistaken for an enthesophyte or avulsion fracture. However, often its increased prominence is the result of bone loss on either side of the crest at the

---

Summary points

- Areas of fiber disruption will have decreased echogenicity regardless of beam angle.
- Areas of scarring will be echogenic regardless of beam angle.
- Dorsal-margin defects and focal enlargement are best identified when the ultrasound beam is not perpendicular to the SL fibers.
- Diffuse mild decreases in echogenicity, especially in the dorsal aspect of the SL, should be interpreted with caution; they are commonly encountered in sound horses and may be the result of relaxation artifact.
- Recheck examination 2 to 4 weeks following initial diagnosis can sometimes reveal worsening of the injury. This initial recheck should be used to plan additional recheck examinations, and may alter the treatment and rehabilitation plan.

---

attachment of the one of the lobes of the SL. The axial margins of the second and fourth metacarpal/tarsal bones and their relationship to the SL should be assessed. As previously mentioned, it is important to remember that placing the carpus in flexion and applying pressure to the palmar soft tissues can change the relationship between the SL and the axial margins of the second and fourth metacarpal bones. The false appearance of contact between a metacarpal bone and the SL can be created with pressure. However, in cases with axial margin proliferation is it important to carefully evaluate the SL margin and fibers for injury. Attempting to position the ultrasound beam perpendicular to the margin adjacent to the bone proliferation will facilitate the identification of injury in this region.

In all cases, comparison with the opposite leg is imperative. In many cases bilateral disease is present. However, one limb is often more affected than the other, so comparison of limbs can still be beneficial. When possible the SL should be reexamined 2 to 4 weeks following the initial diagnosis. In certain cases the injury will be worse in this time frame, despite treatment. Additional rechecks and treatment plans can be made by visualizing the full extent of injury, which should be evident with the combination of these two US examinations.

ADVANCED IMAGING: CT AND MRI

Advanced imaging can be necessary to obtain a diagnosis of SL injury. In certain cases evidence of SL disease is present on high- field MR images, and this disease does not affect the echogenicity enough to make it discernible with US.[11] MRI detects changes in the magnetic properties of the ligament, whereas US detects changes in the acoustic properties. Therefore, MRI will better demonstrate certain types of abnormalities (**Fig. 10**). It is possible that Clinically significant abnormalities can be present in the SL that do not necessarily affect the linearity of the fibers, therefore creating relatively normal US images and abnormal MR images. Subtle abnormalities in the size and shape of the PSL will be more easily detected with MRI. An additional advantage of MRI it that is allows identification of fluid in bone, which is important when evaluating the proximal metacarpal or metatarsal region for evidence of SL injury. Abnormal stress at the SL attachment on the third metacarpal/tarsal bone can cause fluid to accumulate in the bone, resulting in clinical signs without abnormalities in the ligament (**Fig. 11**). MRI is the only method that allows a definitive diagnosis in this case. Nuclear scintigraphy will often have increased IRU in the proximal aspect of the third metacarpal bone in these cases. However, the actual source of the IRU cannot be determined without further imaging. The complex anatomy of the SL makes diagnosis of

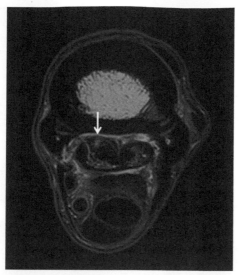

Fig. 10. A focal area of injury is present in the medial lobe of the PSL with increased signal intensity on proton density images. This area did not have concurrent increased signal intensity on fat suppressed images. The diffuse enlargement of the medial lobe of the PSL was evident with ultrasound. However, the focal area of injury in the medial lobe (*arrow*) was echogenic and did not detectably change with alterations in the ultrasound beam angle. Certain types of PSL injury will require MRI for a definitive diagnosis.

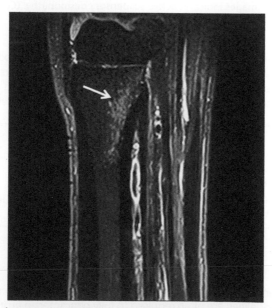

Fig. 11. A sagittal short-tau inversion recovery (STIR) MR image of the proximal metacarpal region. There is fluid in the proximal palmar aspect of the third metacarpal bone at the attachment of the SL (*arrow*). No abnormalities were identified in the SL. Injury to this region resulting in fluid can have corresponding IRU on skeletal scintigraphy examination. However, fluid cannot be differentiated from sclerosis or bone turnover as a source of IRU on a scintigraphy examination. MRI is the only modality that can definitively identify fluid in bone.

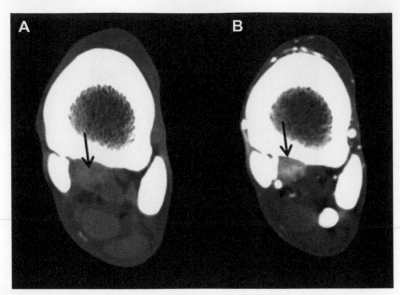

Fig. 12. Precontrast (*A*) and postcontrast (*B*) CT images of a proximal hind suspensory ligament. These images are made at the level of the attachment to the third metatarsal bone. The suspensory ligament is enlarged with loss of the normal fat pattern in the medial aspect of the ligament on the precontrast image (*A*). Furthermore, the ligament appears brighter (hyperattenuating) in this region (*arrow*). In the postcontrast image (*B*), contrast enhancement is present in the medial aspect of the ligament, most prominent dorsally (*arrow*). The appearance on these images indicates active suspensory desmopathy. (*Courtesy of* Sarah M. Puchalski, DVM, DACVR Davis, CA.)

injury using standing MRI challenging. CT can provide information about SL injury, and specifically can evaluate blood flow using intravascular administration of contrast (**Fig. 12**). CT has shorter anesthesia times, but cannot detect fluid in bone and will have decreased sensitivity for soft-tissue lesions when compared with MRI.

Summary points

- Advanced imaging may be required to achieve a diagnosis in cases that have lameness localized to the proximal metacarpal or metatarsal regions and negative radiography, US, and/or nuclear scintigraphy studies.
- Advanced imaging can provide a diagnosis in cases that present as a PSL injury, but have injury in adjacent osseous and/or soft-tissue structures.

SUMMARY

Injury to the SL is an important source of lameness. Because of the complex anatomy of the SL, multiple modalities are often required to fully characterize an injury. A complete US examination of the SL requires different approaches to the ligament and variations in beam angle. This complete US examination will truly represent the anatomy correctly and aid in the differentiation of the complex anatomy from regions of pathologic change. Advanced imaging will be required to detect certain types of injury, and MRI is the only imaging modality that can definitively detect fluid in bone at the SL attachment.

REFERENCES

1. Marks D, Mackay-Smith M, Leslie A, et al. Lameness resulting from high suspensory disease (HSD) in the horse. Proc Am Assoc Equine Pract 1981;24:493–7.
2. Personett L, McAllister S, Mansmann R. Proximal suspensory desmitis. Mod Vet Prac 1983;64:541–5.
3. Pleasant R, Baker G, Muhlbauer M, et al. Stress reactions and stress fractures of the proximal palmar aspect of the third metacarpal bone in horses: 58 cases (1980-1990). J Am Vet Med Assoc 1992;201:1918–23.
4. Bramlage L, Gabel A, Hackett R. Avulsion fracture of the origin of the SL in the horse. J Am Vet Med Assoc 1980;176:1004–10.
5. Denoix JM, Audigie F. Imaging of the musculoskeletal system in horses. In: Hinchcliff KW, Kaneps AJ, Geor RF, editors. Equine sports medicine and surgery. Basic and clinical sciences of the equine athlete. Philadelphia: WB Saunders Co; 2004. p. 161–87.
6. Bischofberger AS, Konar M, Ohlerth S, et al. Magnetic resonance imaging, ultrasonography and histology of the suspensory ligament origin: a comparative study of normal anatomy of Warmblood horses. Equine Vet J 2006;38:508–16.
7. Sisson S. Equine syndesmology. In: Getty R, editor. Sisson and Grossman's anatomy of domestic animals, vol. 1, 5th edition. Philadelphia: WB Saunders; 1975. p. 349–75.
8. Pharr J, Nyland T. Sonography of the equine palmar metacarpal soft tissues of the horse. Equine Vet J 1993;25:30–5.
9. Denoix JM, Coudry V, Jacquet S. Ultrasonographic procedure for a complete examination of the proximal third interosseous muscle in the equine forelimbs. Equine Vet Educ 2008;20:148–53.
10. Denoix JM, Farres D. Ultrasonographic imaging of the proximal third interosseous muscle in the pelvic limb using a plantaromedial approach. J Equine Vet Sci 1995;15(8):346–50.
11. Schramme M, Josson A, Linder K. Characterization of the origin and body of the normal equine rear suspensory ligament using ultrasonography, magnetic resonance imaging, and histology. Vet Radiol Ultrasound 2012;53:318–28.

Advances in Nuclear Medicine

Kurt Selberg, MS, DVM[a],*, Michael Ross, DVM, DACVS[b]

KEYWORDS

- Nuclear Scintigraphy • Equine • Advances • Interpretation

KEY POINTS

- Nuclear scintigraphy (bone scan) is an invaluable tool to aid in the diagnosis in equine lameness.
- Nuclear scintigraphy is highly sensitive for bone injury. However, with this modality there are false-negatives as well as false-positives.
- Advances in software and hardware continue to drive the progress of nuclear scintigraphy.
- Establishing a systematic review of the images helps facilitate more accurate diagnoses.
- A thorough physical and lameness evaluation using diagnostic analgesia is imperative to get the most clinical benefit from a nuclear scintigraphy examination.

INTRODUCTION

Nuclear scintigraphy, specifically bone scintigraphy, is one of the mainstays of molecular imaging. It has preserved its relevance in the imaging of acute and chronic trauma, and is particularly useful in the evaluation of athletic injuries. In the first part of the twentieth century, the relationship between musculoskeletal disorders and accumulation of radioactive substance was first recognized.[1,2] Major advances in technetium-labeled bone tracers were first introduced in 1971.[3] The equine community was introduced to nuclear scintigraphy for diagnosing musculoskeletal disorders shortly after.[4] Since then, nuclear scintigraphy has attained widespread use and availability, with most referral hospitals and universities having γ cameras equipped to accommodate horses. Studies continue to be published highlighting the value and use of nuclear scintigraphy despite the availability of other advanced imaging modalities including computed tomography (CT) and magnetic resonance imaging (MRI). This continued experience and clinical correlation of nuclear scinitigraphy has led to a better understanding of the results from scintigraphic studies and more accurate diagnosis. The

[a] Department of Biosciences and Diagnostic imaging, University of Georgia, 501 D. W. Brooks Drive, Athens, GA 30602, USA; [b] Department of Clinical Studies, New Bolton Center, University of Pennsylvania, 382 West Street Road, Kennett Square, PA 19348, USA
* Corresponding author.
E-mail address: selbergdvm@gmail.com

Vet Clin Equine 28 (2012) 527–538
http://dx.doi.org/10.1016/j.cveq.2012.09.004
0749-0739/12/$ – see front matter Published by Elsevier Inc.

most common use for nuclear scintigraphy in the horse is as a diagnostic tool to aid in lameness diagnosis.[5]

A major advantage of nuclear scintigraphy is that, unlike modalities such as radiography, this imaging modality allows for evaluation of physiologic function.[6] However, the inherent spatial resolution is poor, and thus anatomic detail is lost. Although several radionuclides are available and can diagnose pathologic change in virtually any organ system,[7] the most commonly used radionuclide in horses is technetium 99 m (^{99m}Tc) labeled to tracers (pharmaceuticals) that bind to bone. The most common bone tracers are currently methylene diphosphonate (MDP) and hydroxymethylene diphosphonate (HDP), which have faster soft tissue clearance, increased bone/soft tissue ratios, and better image quality than early bone tracers such as polyphosphates. Although both formulations allow for lesion detection, HDP may have better bone uptake.[8] A bone scan consists of 3 phases after intravenous injection of radiopharmaceutical. The vascular phase (flow phase) occurs within 30 seconds after injection; the soft tissue phase (pool phase), in which the region of interest is imaged 3 to 5 minutes after injection; and the bone phase (delayed phase), with images obtained 2 or more hours after injection.[9] Two-dimensional images, called planar images, are obtained based on counts or time.

The pathologic change associated with bone trauma or injury at a bone-ligament interface (enthesis) results in uptake of bone-seeking radiopharmaceuticals. It is the ability of bone scintigraphy to image the skeleton[5,10–13] that makes it an appealing imaging choice for horses. This ability allows detection of unsuspected sites of trauma that are not recognized in other imaging modalities such as radiography.[14] In addition, nuclear scintigraphy has been reported to be similar in accuracy to MRI for detection of certain bone diseases such as stress fractures in people.[14] This article reviews advances in nuclear scintigraphy and discusses brief principles of, indications for, and limitations of nuclear scintigraphy.

ADVANCES IN EQUIPMENT

Advances in instrumentation have driven increased use of diagnostic imaging in the clinical setting. γ Camera or γ ray scintillation was first developed in 1950,[15] and became commercially available in the 1970s. Despite advances in camera technology and displays, radiotracers still primarily reflect function with limited anatomic resolution.[6] Fine anatomic detail is lost, which can be critical to differentiating physiologic from pathologic change. Advances have been made in combining (fusing) anatomic and physiologic imaging, such as positron emission tomography (PET) combined with CT (PET-CT). These technologies have greatly increased specificity in people for skeletal disease processes.[16,17]

The positron emitter fluorine-18 sodium fluoride was introduced more than 40 years ago as a bone imaging radionuclide. However, it was quickly replaced by ^{99m}Tc because ^{99m}Tc is more readily available, less expensive, and the half-life (6 hours) is advantageous for equine imaging. There is now rapidly increasing availability in human medicine of PET imaging systems; however, sodium fluoride is used instead of ^{99m}Tc. Sodium fluoride has benefits compared with ^{99m}Tc in that it has a 2-fold higher bone uptake and results in a higher target/background ratio.[18] These studies have faster imaging times, better image quality, and more conspicuous lesions, which results in targeted treatment of the disease processes.

The imaging modality PET-CT, although still in its infancy in veterinary medicine and currently unavailable for equine imaging, has integrated well into small animal imaging, specifically oncology studies for staging small animal companions (**Fig. 1**).[19,20] The

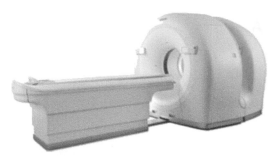

Fig. 1. A positron emission and CT unit. The current design involves the CT inline with the positron emission camera component behind. The current bore size of CT units does not accommodate the body of the equine patient.

current design (**Fig. 2**) of PET systems requires an anatomic imaging system such as CT in line with the positron emission imaging system. Costs for maintaining the infrastructure for PET scans remain high.[21]

The combination of scintigraphy and CT allows for earlier detection of bone abnormalities compared with radiography and plain CT, but is similar to that of MRI.[22] Another application, single-positron emission CT (SPECT), uses ^{99m}Tc and information is acquired and reconstructed to obtain three-dimensional images. Advances in γ camera design have made it possible to acquire volumetric data sets, thus giving cross-sectional images. As with PET, these images may be fused with anatomic imaging such as CT. In people, the addition of fused images with SPECT increases diagnostic confidence compared with planar scintigraphic and regular CT images.[17] The current designs for SPECT/CT fusions are similar to PET imaging, requiring a γ camera in line with CT. Even without fusion with anatomic studies, in human diagnostic imaging, cross-sectional bone scan (single-positron emission) images have a greater sensitivity for osseous lesions compared with planar bone scan images.[23] CT of the equine distal limb is currently available.[24] With advances in technology and innovative design, SPECT fused with CT may be a future direction of nuclear imaging in horses, but is currently not available.

FUNDAMENTALS OF CONVENTIONAL NUCLEAR SCINTIGRAPHY

Planar (two-dimensional imaging) bone scintigraphy remains simple and easy to perform. The basic concept of the γ camera has not changed in the last 50 years.[25] This design incorporates a thallium-doped sodium iodine crystal that scintillates in response to γ photons (rays). This scintillation in turn produces a small flash of light that is transferred to photomultiplier tubes that detect the flash. The photon resolution is limited by the physical characteristics of the sodium iodide crystal and photomultiplier. The spatial resolution is reduced by the collimator and number of photomultipliers.[26]

Solid-state γ cameras have recently been developed with increased sensitivity as well as spatial resolution, which is performed using semiconductors to detect γ rays. Semiconductors directly produce electron currents in response to γ photons, and combine the functions of scintillation crystal and photomultiplier tubes. Semiconductor systems use cadmium-zinc-telluride for photon detection[26] rather than a sodium iodine crystal, and directly convert a photon to a digital signal. This results in signal precision that is better than that of scintillators, resulting in correspondingly better energy resolution.[27] These systems are less bulky and weigh around 150 kg.

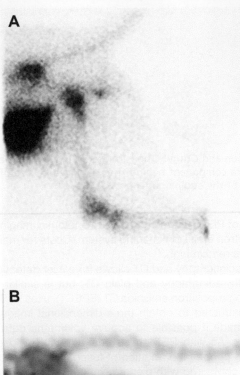

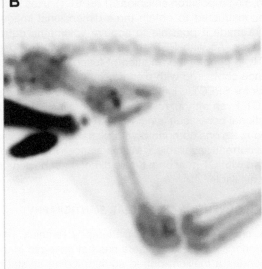

Fig. 2. Left lateral images of a canine pelvis and femur. (*A*) Planar technetium 99m image. (*B*) Planar image of the same patient using sodium fluoride as the radiotracer. There is greater bone uptake and higher target/background ratio in the sodium fluoride scan compared with technetium images.

The disadvantage is a smaller field of view and higher fabrication cost compared with conventional γ cameras.

ADVANCES IN SOFTWARE

Many advances in nuclear medicine have come in the form of software. Because nuclear scintigraphy for the most part is performed on a standing, sedated horse, acquisition stations are equipped with the ability to account for motion, known as dynamic capture. In addition, region-of-interest calculation, line-profile analysis, algorithms to filter noise, and attenuation correction to account for variation between images are available.

Motion correct improves the image quality in examinations of the standing sedated horse. This process obtains images at 1-second to 2-second intervals that are stacked. The outlying images from excessive motion (spatial misregistration) are rejected. The images within the same spatial registration are superimposed on one another, creating an image with better resolution compared with single, static acquisitions. The software correction is particularly useful when imaging the axial skeleton (**Fig. 3**), which is evident in the spine and pelvis where areas of abnormal

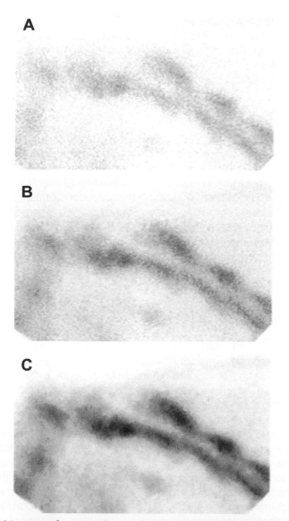

Fig. 3. Left lateral images of a normal cranial cervical spine. (*A*) The image (148 K) has too few counts and decreased signal/noise. (*B*) The image (250 K) has good signal/noise and good anatomic definition. (*C*) A filter to decrease noise and increase signal has been applied to the 148-K image. There is now good signal/noise.

radiopharmaceutical uptake may not be visible on uncorrected images.[28] Compared with uncorrected images, motion-corrected images are clearer and the anatomy is more distinct. However, the technique has limitations when motion is excessive.[29]

Quantitative analysis can be performed routinely using most nuclear medicine software programs. For instance, a region of interest (ROI) can be outlined and a numerical value assigned and compared with the contralateral anatomic area. Although subjective scoring correlates well with quantitative scores in scintigraphic studies,[30] subtle differences or abnormal radiopharmaceutical uptake may be more readily identified by using ROI analysis.[28] Count differences of specific ROIs can be calculated and background counts can be normalized.[5] However, when using ROI analysis, care must be taken that the region is of clinical importance and relevant to the case.[28]

Most nuclear medicine software can analyze images using algorithms that are designed to remove artifact or noise and increase signal to improve image quality. Using these computer algorithms to filter noise can be particularly useful when subtle pathologic change is present or if adequate counts cannot be obtained because of patient disposition (see **Fig. 3**).[31] Use of filters designed to increase signal and filter noise tend to make areas of increased radiopharmaceutical uptake more obvious.[11] However, at higher counts, an increased rate of false-positives may occur.[31]

INDICATIONS AND LIMITATIONS

There are many indications for use nuclear scintigraphy as a diagnostic aid. These indications vary with the phase of bone scan. Pool phase images, which allow for examination of the soft tissues, should be considered for horses with acute lameness, after trauma, or in cases in which soft tissue uptake would alter the diagnosis. Hyperemia, characterized by abnormal radiopharmaceutical uptake, is evident in the affected tissues. Delayed uptake is present only if there is necrosis or calcification, or the affected tissue is in close proximity to adjacent bony structures.[32] Indications for bone or pool phase imaging include acute or chronic lameness, obscure or multilimb lameness, poor performance, lameness that is localized to a specific region but other imaging fails to reveal abnormalities, and anatomic regions that are difficult to evaluate with other imaging modalities.[5,9,33,34]

INTERPRETATION PRINCIPLES

A systematic approach to interpreting images should be used. Symmetry between right and left, pattern, and intensity of uptake are assessed and correlated with anatomy to determine an appropriate differential diagnosis. Evaluating the images in the same order is also recommended to avoid missing views. Abnormal radiopharmaceutical uptake is typically assessed as focal or diffuse. Focal increased radiopharmaceutical uptake is generally thought to be confined to a specific anatomic location such as abnormality at the insertion of a ligament/tendon or may indicate the presence of a stress or traumatic fracture. Diffuse uptake of radiopharmaceutical indicates that an area of increased radiopharmaceutical uptake is more widespread. For instance, focal, moderate to intense increased radiopharmaceutical uptake in the dorsal cortex of the third metacarpal bone suggests a dorsal cortical fracture, whereas diffuse increased radiopharmaceutical uptake involving most of the cortex indicates that the horse has periostitis. Increased radiopharmaceutical uptake is judged from mild to intense. In general, there is good correlation between severity of clinical signs and radiopharmaceutical uptake. However, focal areas void of radiopharmaceutical uptake (photopenia) may also be regions of pathologic change. This change is a result

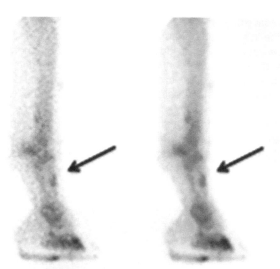

Fig. 4. Right forelimb of a 10-year-old Warmblood jumper with no apparent front limb lameness. There is focal, mild-to-moderate, radiopharmaceutical uptake in the mid-dorsal aspect of the proximal phalanx (*arrows*). On the left is a static image with 200 k counts, and the image on the right is a filtered image to increase signal and reduce noise.

of decreased or absent blood flow. Specific disorders resulting in photopenia include infectious osteitis, bone sequestrum, and thrombus.[35]

Increased radiopharmaceutical uptake reflects an area of bone turnover or bone modeling (formation), and may neither be pathologic nor of clinical relevance.[11] The physes of young horses have marked increased uptake, in particular the distal radial physis, and may continue to have uptake beyond radiological closure.[36,37] Because radiopharmaceutical uptake can normally be intense in physeal regions, adjacent pathologic changes, if small or subtle, may be obscured on the bone scan images

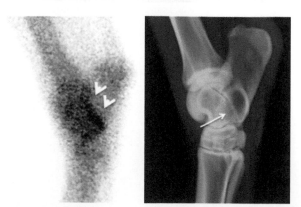

Fig. 5. Lateral scintigraphic image of the left tarsus and lateromedial radiograph image of the left tarsus. There is moderate linear radiopharmaceutical uptake in the region of the ta-localcaneal joint (*arrowheads*). The radiopharmaceutical uptake in the region of the distal intertarsal joint and tarsometatarsal joint is within normal limits. There is focal osteolysis and irregularity along the mediodistal aspect of the talocalcaneal joint (*arrow*). The distal intertarsal joint is narrowed; however, subchondral bone is not sclerotic and thickened.

because normal active physes steal counts from important or relevant areas nearby. In the absence of the intense radiopharmaceutical uptake from the physis, these more subtle regions become evident. In addition, abnormal radiopharmaceutical uptake may be associated with athletic events without clinical relevance (**Fig. 4**).[38,39] When horses return to or just start work, increase radiopharmaceutical uptake may similarly be present in the distal metacarpal/tarsal subchondral bone without associated lameness.[30]

Nuclear medicine is useful for directing the focus and critical evaluation of a particular anatomic area. Tarsal osteoarthropathies are a common site of pathologic change, especially in the distal intertarsal and tarsometatarsal joints.[40] Although radiological abnormalities are also common, these may not reflect a source of pain causing

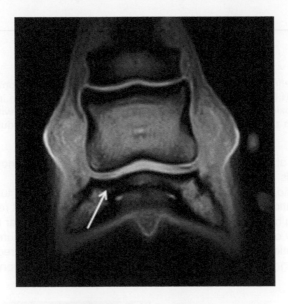

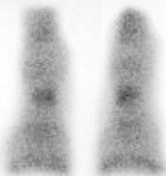

Fig. 6. T1-weighted, gradient-echo, dorsal plane image of the left forefoot and concurrent dorsal nuclear scintigraphic images. Lateral is to the right on the magnetic resonance image. There is subchondral bone sclerosis of the medial aspect of the distal phalanx (*arrow*) characterized by low signal (*black*). There was concurrent low signal on short tau inversion recovery images. The dorsal image of the distal aspect of the forelimbs has uniform and symmetric radiopharmaceutical uptake in the mid-dorsal aspect of the phalanges.

lameness.[41] Obscure locations of pathologic change may be more relevant, despite concurrent radiological abnormalities present in common locations, such as the distal joints of the tarsus (**Fig. 5**).

False-negative scintigraphic findings can occur. Medial femoral condyle cysts, although increasing in size radiologically, may not exhibit increased radiopharmaceutical uptake on caudal images.[42] It is proposed that bone undergoing resorption from osteoclastic activity without osteoblastic activity would not deposit new matrix and could remain scintigraphically quiescent.[42] Although scintigraphically normal, intra-articular analgesia confirmed that the source of pain causing lameness was the stifle in the horse included in that study. Osteosclerosis in the distal phalanx similarly may have a normal scintigraphic pattern of uptake (**Fig. 6**), which may also be the result of minimal osteoblastic activity with little new bone matrix. However, nuclear scintigraphy may be a useful tool to follow healing of osteochondrosis lesions and return to normal activity levels.[43]

Increased radiopharmaceutical uptake may also be noted globally in the contralateral limb secondary to aberrant weight bearing. This observation is particularly evident in the dorsal/plantar images, in which both limbs are present in a single image (**Fig. 7**). Asymmetry has previously been observed in the metacarpal and metatarsal regions of horses with no appreciable lameness, and may reflect preferential limb use.[44] In contrast, horses that had a limb immobilized in a cast may have increased radiopharmaceutical uptake following cast removal, possibly caused by normal adaptation, a pathologic response to immobilization, and/or remobilization.[45]

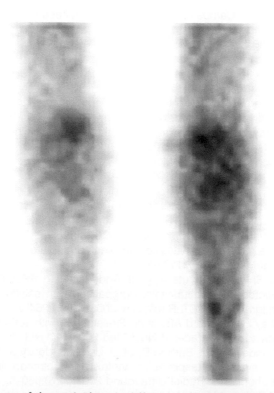

Fig. 7. Plantar image of the tarsi. There is diffuse, moderate radiopharmaceutical present throughout the crus, tarsus, and metatarsal bones of the right hind, the nonlame limb.

SUMMARY

Many advances in nuclear scintigraphic imaging have made the modality a remarkable diagnostic tool. Nuclear scintigraphy is highly sensitive for bone injury,[46–51] but there are false-negatives as well as false-positives. Thus, a thorough physical, lameness evaluation, and diagnostic analgesia are key to getting the most from a nuclear scintigraphic scan.

REFERENCES

1. Blum T. Osteomyelitis of the mandible and maxilla. J Am Dent Assoc 1924;11: 802–5.
2. Martland AA. Osteogenic sarcoma in dial painters using luminous paint. Arch Pathol 1929;7:406–17.
3. McAfee GS. A new complex of 99mTc for skeletal imaging. Radiology 1971;99: 192–6.
4. Ueltschi G. Bone and joint imaging with 99mTc labelled phosphates as a new diagnostic aid in veterinary orthopedics. Vet Radiol Ultrasound 1977;18(3):80–9.
5. Archer DC, Boswell JC, Voute LC, et al. Skeletal scintigraphy in the horse: current indications and validity as a diagnostic test. Vet J 2007;173(1):31–44.
6. Weaver MP. Twenty years of equine scintigraphy–a coming of age? Equine Vet J 1995;27(3):163–5.
7. Hornof WJ, Koblik PD. The scintigraphic detection of muscle damage. Equine Vet J 1991;23(5):327–8.
8. Arndt J, Pauwels E, Camps J, et al. Clinical differences between bone-seeking agents. Eur J Nucl Med 1985;11(8):330.
9. Lamb C, Koblik P. Scintigraphic evaluation of skeletal disease and its application to the horse. Vet Radiol Ultrasound 1988;29(1):16–27.
10. Dyson S. Sixteen fractures of the shoulder region in the horse. Equine Vet J 1985; 17(2):104–10.
11. Dyson SJ. Subjective and quantitative scintigraphic assessment of the equine foot and its relationship with foot pain. Equine Vet J 2002;34(2):164–70.
12. Dyson S, Murray R. Pain associated with the sacroiliac joint region: a clinical study of 74 horses. Equine Vet J 2003;35(3):240–5.
13. Smith RK, Dyson SJ, Schramme MC, et al. Osteoarthritis of the talocalcaneal joint in 18 horses. Equine Vet J 2005;37(2):166–71.
14. Van der Wall H, Lee A, Magee M, et al. Radionuclide bone scintigraphy in sports injuries. Semin Nucl Med 2010;40(1):16–30.
15. Anger HO. Scintillation camera. Rev Sci Instrum 1958;29:27–33.
16. Romer W, Nomayr A, Uder M, et al. SPECT-guided CT for evaluating foci of increased bone metabolism classified as an intermediate on SPECT in cancer patients. J Nucl Med 2006;47:1102–6.
17. Utsunomiya D, Shiraishi S, Imuta M, et al. Added value of SPECT/CT fusion in assessing suspected bone metastasis: comparison with scintigraphy alone and nonfused scintigraphy and CT. Radiology 2006;238(1):264–71.
18. Grant FD, Fahey FH, Packard AB, et al. Skeletal PET with 18F-fluoride: applying new technology to an old tracer. J Nucl Med 2008;49(1):68–78.
19. Lawrence J, Vanderhoek M, Barbee D, et al. Use of 3'-deoxy-3'[18F] fluorothymidine PET/CT for evaluating response to cytotoxic chemotherapy in dogs with non-Hodgkin's lymphoma. Vet Radiol Ultrasound 2009;50(6):660–8.
20. Lee MS, Lee AR, Jung MA, et al. Characterization of physiologic 18F-FDG uptake with PET-CT in dogs. Vet Radiol Ultrasound 2010;51(6):670–3.

21. Peremans K, Cornelissen B, Van Den Bossche B, et al. Review of small animal imaging planar and pinhole spect γ camera imaging. Vet Radiol Ultrasound 2005;46(2):162–70.
22. Palestro CJ, Love C, Schneider R. The evolution of nuclear medicine and the musculoskeletal system. Radiol Clin North Am 2009;47(3):505–32.
23. Minoves M. Bone and joint sports injuries: the role of bone scintigraphy. Nucl Med Commun 2003;24(1):3–10.
24. Desbrosse FG, Vandeweerd JM, Perrin RA, et al. A technique for computed tomography (CT) of the foot in the standing horse. Equine Vet Educ 2008;20(2):93–8.
25. Anger HO. Scintillation camera with multichannel collimators. J Nucl Med 1964;5: 515–31.
26. Sharir T, Slomka PJ, Berman DS. Solid-state SPECT technology: fast and furious. J Nucl Cardiol 2010;17(5):890–6.
27. Madsen MT. Recent advances in SPECT imaging. J Nucl Med 2007;48(4): 661–73.
28. Davenport-Goodall CL, Ross MW. Scintigraphic abnormalities of the pelvic region in horses examined because of lameness or poor performance: 128 cases (1993-2000). J Am Vet Med Assoc 2004;224(1):88–95.
29. Dyson S, Murray R, Branch M, et al. The sacroiliac joints: evaluation using nuclear scintigraphy. Part 1: the normal horse. Equine Vet J 2003;35(3):226–32.
30. Kawcak C, McIlwraith C, Norrdin R, et al. Clinical effects of exercise on subchondral bone of carpal and metacarpophalangeal joints in horses. Am J Vet Res 2000;61(10):1252–8.
31. Eksell P, Carlsson S, Lord P, et al. Effects of a digital filter on detectability of a phantom lesion in a scintigram of the equine tarsus. Vet Radiol Ultrasound 2000;41(4):365–70.
32. Van der Wall H, Fogelman I. Scintigraphy of benign bone disease. Semin Musculoskelet Radiol 2007;11(4):281–300.
33. Davidson E, Ross M. Clinical recognition of stress-related bone injury in racehorses. Clin Tech Equine Pract 2003;2(4):296–311.
34. Hoskinson J. Equine nuclear scintigraphy - indications, uses, and techniques. Vet Clin North Am Equine Pract 2001;17(1):63–74.
35. Levine DG, Ross BM, Ross MW, et al. Decreased radiopharmaceutical uptake (photopenia) in delayed phase scintigraphic images in three horses. Vet Radiol Ultrasound 2007;48(5):467–70.
36. Uhlhorn H, Eksell P, Carlsten J. Scintigraphic characterization of distal radial physeal closure in young standardbred racehorses. Vet Radiol Ultrasound 2000;41(2):181–6.
37. Twardock AR. Equine bone scintigraphic uptake patterns related to age, breed, and occupation. Vet Clin North Am Equine Pract 2001;17(1):75–94.
38. Bailey RE, Dyson SJ, Parkin TD. Focal increased radiopharmaceutical uptake in the dorsoproximal diaphyseal region of the equine proximal phalanx. Vet Radiol Ultrasound 2007;48(5):460–6.
39. Ehrlich PJ, Seeherman HJ, O'Callaghan MW, et al. Results of bone scintigraphy in horses used for show jumping, hunting, or eventing: 141 cases (1988-1994). J Am Vet Med Assoc 1998;213(10):1460–7.
40. Dabareiner RM, Cohen ND, Carter GK, et al. Musculoskeletal problems associated with lameness and poor performance among horses used for barrel racing: 118 cases (2000-2003). J Am Vet Med Assoc 2005;227(10):1646–50.
41. Fairburn A, Dyson S, Murray R. Clinical significance of osseous spurs on the dorsoproximal aspect of the third metatarsal bone. Equine Vet J 2010;42(7):591–9.

42. Squire KR, Fessler JF, Cantwell HD, et al. Enlarging bilateral femoral condylar bone cysts without scintigraphic uptake in a yearling foal. Vet Radiol Ultrasound 1992;33(2):109–13.
43. Cahill BR, Berg BC. 99m-Technetium phosphate compound joint scintigraphy in the management of juvenile osteochondritis dissecans of the femoral condyles. Am J Sports Med 1983;11(5):329–35.
44. Weekes JS, Murray RC, Dyson SJ. Scintigraphic evaluation of metacarpophalangeal and metatarsophalangeal joints in clinically sound horses. Vet Radiol Ultrasound 2004;45(1):85–90.
45. Van Harreveld PD, Lillich JD, Kawcak CE, et al. Clinical evaluation of the effects of immobilization followed by remobilization and exercise on the metacarpophalangeal joint in horses. Am J Vet Res 2002;63(2):282–8.
46. Pleasant RS, Baker GJ, Muhlbauer MC, et al. Stress reactions and stress fractures of the proximal palmar aspect of the third metacarpal bone in horses: 58 cases (1980-1990). J Am Vet Med Assoc 1992;201(12):1918–23.
47. O'Sullivan CB, Lumsden JM. Stress fractures of the tibia and humerus in thoroughbred racehorses: 99 cases (1992-2000). J Am Vet Med Assoc 2003; 222(4):491–8.
48. Mackey VS, Trout DR, Meagher DM, et al. Stress fractures of the humerus, radius, and tibia in horses. Vet Radiol Ultrasound 1987;28(1):26–31.
49. Nelson A. Stress fractures of the hind limb in 2 thoroughbreds. Equine Vet Educ 1994;6:245–8.
50. Davidson EJ, Martin BB Jr. Stress fracture of the scapula in two horses. Vet Radiol Ultrasound 2004;45(5):407–10.
51. Koblik PD, Hornof WJ, Seeherman HJ. Scintigraphic appearance of stress-induced trauma of the dorsal cortex of the third metacarpal bone in racing thoroughbred horses: 121 cases (1978-1986). J Am Vet Med Assoc 1988;192(3): 390–5.

Musculoskeletal Injury in Thoroughbred Racehorses
Correlation of Findings Using Multiple Imaging Modalities

Lorrie Gaschen, PhD, DVM, Dr Med Vet*, Daniel J. Burba, DVM

KEYWORDS

- Stress remodeling • Adaptive • Sclerosis • MRI • Bone scans

KEY POINTS

- Radiography is an important modality for many osseous injuries and fractures but is unreliable for diagnosing acute nondisplaced fractures and subtle subchondral bone disorders.
- Bone scintigraphy is a highly sensitive diagnostic imaging modality for identifying subchondral bone injury and stress-related bone remodeling and fractures. However, because this modality reflects physiology, it is nonspecific for differentiating among discrete types of pathologic change.
- MRI examination is able to show adaptive and nonadaptive bone remodeling that is radiographically silent in Thoroughbred racehorses. Subchondral bone damage is often characterized by increased signal intensity on fat-suppressed images bordered by low signal intensity of the plantar or palmar aspect of the distal third metatarsal and third metacarpal in T1-weighted, T2-weighted, and proton density sequences. This pattern is often representative of osteonecrosis that is bordered by sclerosis.
- Fluid in bone can be diagnosed with MRI, and is caused by many pathologic processes, including hemorrhage, necrosis, and edema. The characteristic signal pattern consists of intraosseous hyperintensity on T2-weighted, short-tau inversion recovery, or fat-suppressed MRI images.
- Ultrasonography is the most common preferred modality for examining flexor tendon and suspensory apparatus diseases. However, MRI may be superior for assessing ligament injury in the pastern and subcarpal region. Soft tissue injuries may require both modalities for complete evaluation.

The authors have nothing to disclose.
Department of Veterinary Clinical Sciences, Louisiana State University, Skip Bertman Drive, Baton Rouge, LA 70803, USA
* Corresponding author.
E-mail address: lgaschen@lsu.edu

INTRODUCTION

Imaging of musculoskeletal disease in Thoroughbred racehorses has historically relied on radiography and ultrasound to diagnose fractures, osteoarthritis, and soft tissue injuries. Scintigraphy has been traditionally used to screen for regions of increased radiopharmaceutical uptake (IRU) to direct radiographic examinations and diagnose acute disease that may be radiographically silent. Current research is now focused on the imaging of adaptive and nonadaptive stress-related diseases and has led to the greater understanding of sources of pain and why catastrophic fractures occur. Most fetlock lameness is caused by subchondral bone disease that cannot be appreciated radiographically until osteophytes, osteochondral fragments, subchondral bone lysis, or fractures occur later in the course of the disease process. Osteochondral fragmentation and fracture, subchondral bone necrosis, and osteoarthritis are common diseases in athletic horses, and subchondral bone plays an integral role in the pathogenesis of these diseases.[1] In addition to fractures, marked subchondral bone sclerosis and joint damage are common in young racehorses.[2]

IMAGING OF ADAPTIVE AND NONADAPTIVE PROCESSES IN THE THOROUGHBRED RACEHORSE

The following is a definition of terms that will be used in this section:

- Modeling: bone formation and resorption to produce functionally and mechanically purposeful architecture.
- Remodeling: absorption of abnormal bone tissue and simultaneous deposition of new bone; in normal bone, modeling and remodeling are in dynamic equilibrium.
- Adaptive change: the process of modeling and remodeling of bone in response to forces applied to it over time.
- Nonadaptive change: the rate of bone removal (absorption) exceeds the rate of bone replacement, weakening the bone and making it more susceptible to injury such as stress fractures.

Many anatomic regions in the Thoroughbred racehorse can be a source of lameness. Pathologic evidence indicates that most osseous injuries are repetitive overuse injuries (stress-related bone injury). Evidence of stress remodeling is observed in association with fracture interfaces of equine long, cuboidal, and irregular bones.[3]

Adaptive changes of osseous structures involve the process of modeling and remodeling. Modeling is defined as bone formation and resorption to produce functionally and mechanically purposeful architecture. Remodeling occurs when damaged bone is replaced.[1,4] In the optimal stress and strain environment, bone formation and resorption are quiescent. Bone resorption occurs below the minimum strain threshold, and bone formation occurs above the maximum. Subchondral bone density and strength adapt to stresses.

The third carpal bone (C3) and palmar aspect of the third metacarpal (McIII) and third metatarsal (MtIII) condyles of horses often undergo modeling and remodeling in racehorses. These bones can increase in density in response to training and can eventually become sclerotic.[1,2] This alteration is significant because subchondral bone provides cushioning of the joint, even more than the articular cartilage.[5] However, adaptive and nonadaptive osseous changes in the Thoroughbred racehorse resulting in sclerosis may be associated with only subtle changes in bone density and structure. This occurrence results in slight, if any, changes in radiopacity and is usually best seen on either high-quality single-screen film systems or digital radiography (DR). Furthermore, special radiographic views, bone scintigraphy, CT, and MRI are often necessary to detect subtle changes in bone density and structure of the affected trabecular and subchondral bone.

Racehorses exhibit tremendous changes within the subchondral bone of their metacarpophalangeal and carpal joints. These changes can lead to damage ranging from osteochondral fragmentation to life-threatening catastrophic fractures. The presentation of a racehorse with forelimb lameness localized to the fetlock, proximal metacarpus, or distal carpus with few radiographic or ultrasonographic findings is common.[6] Because of the increased sensitivity of bone scintigraphy and MRI to osseous change, they are important modalities to use in these cases. The extensive variation in the severity of disease present in these highly affected joints requires imaging modalities that can identity a range of injuries, from subtle to severe, to obtain a diagnosis.

Radiography is usually the first imaging modality used once lameness is localized to a specific region, because of its wide availability and the well-established descriptions of most diseases. However, it is unreliable for diagnosing subtle or nondisplaced fractures and certain types or severities of subchondral bone disorders.[7]

Bone scintigraphy is a highly sensitive diagnostic imaging modality for identifying subchondral bone injury and stress-related changes. However, it is nonspecific for defining discrete pathologic abnormalities because it reflects bone physiology and does not provide the anatomic detail achieved with the other imaging modalities.[8] Cortical and subchondral stress-related bone injuries are frequent, and scintigraphic examination is very important to detect their presence. Stress fractures can be present in horses with obscure or undiagnosed lameness. Diagnosis of stress fractures can prevent the development of complete fractures, which often result from having previous stress-related bone injuries in cortical or trabecular bone. Recheck scintigraphic examination is indicated in horses with evidence of stress fractures before they return to work.

MRI examination is able to show adaptive and nonadaptive bone remodeling that is not radiographically evident. Sclerosis is characterized by low signal intensity in the plantar or palmar aspect of the distal MtIII/McIII on T1-weighted, T2-weighted, and proton density (PD) images. Sclerosis identified using MRI can correlate with IRU on scintigraphy examination, and this correlation can be used to determine clinical significance.[9]

Bone marrow–type edema is a term used to describe a characteristic MRI appearance resulting from replacement of bone marrow fat by material containing H+ ions, in the form of water.[6] This term has been established to describe a signal pattern in racehorses that may represent several possible pathophysiologic processes.[6] This characteristic signal pattern consists of intraosseous T2-weighted, short-tau inversion recovery (STIR), and fat-suppressed hyperintensity with corresponding T1-weighted hypointensity (**Fig. 1**).[10]

Increased signal intensity in bone on fat-suppressed images indicates fluid, which can be the result of contusion, stress-related edema, or osteonecrosis. Studies have reported that lesions characterized by hyperintensity in the proximal McIII on fluid-sensitive sequences (STIR and fat-saturated) can be a source of pain caused by a stress reaction through repetitive loading of the proximal metacarpus.[6] These signal alterations as a result of fluid in bone indicate primary osseous pathologic change with minimal involvement of the suspensory ligament.[6] Progression of bone injury appears as high signal intensity on fat-suppressed and inversion recovery images from necrosis, ischemia, and/or edema, and is surrounded by a region of sclerosis.

CT can be used to quantify adaptive changes, such as subchondral bone sclerosis, and for surgical planning of fracture repair. In a study of Thoroughbred racehorses with osteoarthritis, distal metacarpophalangeal condyle sclerosis diagnosed with CT

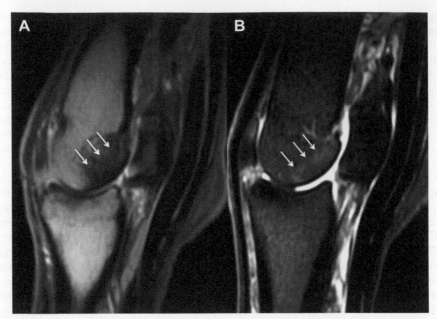

Fig. 1. (*A*) PD and (*B*) short-tau inversion recovery (STIR) parasagittal images of the fetlock showing a hypointense (PD) and hyperintense (STIR) lesion (*arrows*) at the palmar aspect of the metacarpal condyle typical of a subchondral bone damage caused by nonadaptive remodeling in a Thoroughbred racehorse characterized by sclerosis and fluid.

correlated to morphologically thickened trabeculae and lamellar bone formation. The regions of sclerosis on CT were associated with cartilage lesions at the same site and were most severe in the palmar aspect of the condyles.[9] CT shows fracture lines and the extent of the bone damage in much greater detail than radiography, improving the understanding of comminuted fractures.[11]

This article focuses on comparative imaging in Thoroughbred racehorses using radiography, ultrasound, nuclear scintigraphy, CT, and MRI.

METACARPOPHALANGEAL AND METATARSOPHALANGEAL JOINT LAMENESS

The metacarpophalangeal and metatarsophalangeal joints are the focus of several types of injuries, such as subchondral bone pain caused by adaptive and nonadaptive remodeling, osteoarthritis, fractures, and soft tissue injuries. In general, cortical fractures and osteoarthritis are easier to recognize radiographically than stress-related remodeling or fractures of cancellous bone. Most imaging modalities have limitations in the metacarpophalangeal/metatarsophalangeal joint region. Radiography and scintigraphy may not be capable of detecting early cartilage loss and subchondral bone injury without marked structural bone damage or demineralization, and MRI may be necessary for diagnosis.[12,13] High-field MRI is superior to other imaging modalities for assessing articular cartilage and detecting subchondral bone sclerosis. Ultrasonographic evaluation is helpful in the examination of the supporting soft tissue structures of the metacarpophalangeal/metatarsophalangeal joints, but is less sensitive than MRI for certain types of injuries of the straight and oblique distal sesamoidean ligaments.[14–16] Studies examining the use of MRI in the metacarpophalangeal and metatarsophalangeal region have shown that the most common combinations of lesions involve subchondral bone injuries and abnormalities of the suspensory apparatus, and subchondral bone injuries and chondral or osteochondral lesions.[17]

MRI Signal Intensity Pattern of Subchondral and Trabecular Bone Injury

Abnormal signal in the subchondral bone includes (1) diffuse or focal signal increase on STIR images consistent with bone edema, contusion, and bruising or cellular infiltration, (2) focal signal increase in T1-weighted, PD, and T2-weighted sequences associated with loss of trabecular, subchondral, or cortical bone,[17] and (3) diffuse signal decrease in T1-weighted, PD, and T2-weighted sequences indicating increased trabecular density. Osseous hypointensity represents osteosclerosis caused by remodeling in response to chronic bone injury.[17] PD-weighted images are excellent for recognizing sclerosis (**Figs. 2** and **3**). PD-weighted images provide good anatomic detail of bone, including trabecular thickness and density. Concurrent soft tissue injury has been shown to be present in a large percentage of horses with subchondral injury recognized with MRI.[17]

Palmar/Plantar Condyle Disease, Subchondral Bone Sclerosis, and Fractures

Understanding that subchondral bone disease is a substantial cause of lameness but may not manifest itself radiographically is important. Adaptive modeling can progress to nonadaptive remodeling, leading to bone injury of the distal McIII and MtIII bones. Ultimately, subchondral bone damage to the distal McIII and MtIII can lead to fracture and the progression of osteoarthritis. Metacarpal condylar fractures occur at sites that have lost normal trabecular architecture because of localized increased bone

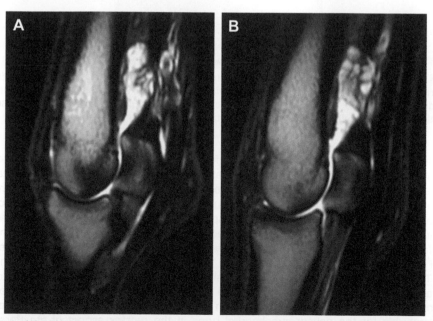

Fig. 2. (A) PD MRI parasagittal image of the medial condyle of the right distal third metacarpus showing hypointensity in the palmar aspect of the condyle representing moderate to severe sclerosis. (B) PD MRI parasagittal image of the lateral condyle of the distal third metacarpus of the same horse as in **Fig. 1A**. Palmar hypointensity caused by mild sclerosis can be seen and compared with the medial condyle in (A).

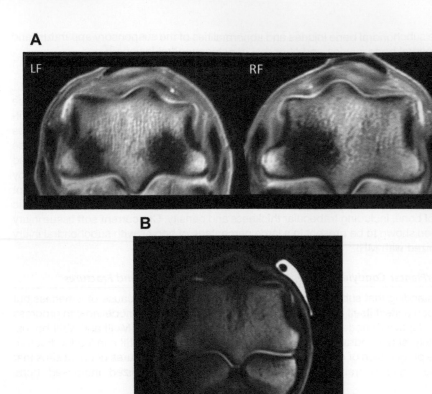

Fig. 3. (*A*) Transverse PD MRI images of the same horse as in **Fig. 1**. The left and right meta-carpal condyles both show parasagittal hypointensity from sclerosis that was not evident radiographically. (*B*) Transverse PD MRI image of the metacarpal condyles of other horse. Although the condyles are normal, focal sagittal ridge sclerosis is present.

volume.[4] Pathologic features of condylar fracture, such as subchondral bone sclerosis, cracking, and erosion, are readily detectable with cross-sectional imaging but often are not radiographically evident. Poor correlation between radiographs and the pathologic change actually present is mainly because of the inability of radiography to adequately isolate the palmar aspect of McIII.[18] CT and MRI are better at detecting subchondral sclerosis compared with radiography.[19] Subchondral bone sclerosis scores with CT and MRI have been shown to correlate well with quantified CT bone mineral density.[19]

The proximal phalanx (P1) in Thoroughbred racehorses has been shown radiographically to develop palmar subchondral bone thickening after training.[20] Hyperextension and extreme load-bearing, which increase with high-speed exercise, are responsible for the denser subchondral bone in the palmar aspect of the P1 as opposed to the dorsal aspect.[20] Furthermore, differences in load-bearing can be appreciated when comparing palmar cortical bone thickness between inside and outside legs of Thoroughbred racehorses after training.[21] Sagittal P1 fractures have been reported as one of the most common fractures of the Thoroughbred racehorse in the United Kingdom, resulting in significant morbidity and occasional mortality.[22] One study compared radiography, scintigraphy, and MRI in 3 horses and found that focal IRU in the proximodorsal aspect of P1 corresponded to a marked bone marrow edema–like signal pattern within the trabecular bone on MR images. These horses had normal radiographic studies that included additional views of the fetlock.[23] It was concluded that the imaging findings were similar to those seen in the distal McIII and MtIII, and are most likely related to stress injury.

Parasagittal fractures of the McIII and MtIII condyles are one of the most common sites of long bone fractures of the Thoroughbred racehorse.[18] Fracture visibility on radiographs depends on fracture extent, displacement, and superimposition of structures. In 22 racehorses with condylar fractures, radiography, CT, and gross appearance were compared.[24] Radiography does not provide complete visualization of the extent of the condylar fractures when compared with cross-sectional imaging modalities such as CT.[24] For most pathologic change, agreement is generally higher between CT and gross examination compared with radiographs because of the superior ability of CT to image McIII and MtIII at the palmar and plantar aspects, respectively. Proximally extending fissure lines in McIII and MtIII are also best detected using CT, and more than 50% of fissures are missed radiographically.[24] CT is especially advantageous for assessing condylar fractures when it can be used immediately before surgery under the same anesthesia.[11]

Palmar osteochondral disease, previously termed *traumatic osteochondrosis*, has been shown to be present in 67% of Thoroughbred racehorses at post mortem, and the distal palmar/plantar McIII/MtIII condyles are the most common sites of IRU in that disease process (see **Fig. 3**).[2,25] Negative radiographs do not eliminate the presence of this disease as a source of pain, and scintigraphy is more sensitive than radiography for detection. Scintigraphic examination reveals focal areas of IRU from adaptive and nonadaptive remodeling or fracture, and better demonstrates the presence of disease because radiographs are often negative.[7] As the disease progresses, radiographic changes can include flattening of the distal McIII/MtIII condyles, sclerosis of the trabecular bone, and radiolucency of the subchondral bone (**Fig. 4**). If the disease is severe, pitting of the subchondral bone with lucency that extends into the trabecular bone can be identified on radiographs. Most subchondral lesions that are identified with MRI correlate with areas of IRU on scintigraphic examination. Furthermore, MRI has often shown subchondral bone lesions to have concurrent soft tissue injuries that may not be evident with other imaging modalities.[17] However, nuclear scintigraphy likely best demonstrates the activity of a bone lesion detected with MRI. Therefore, multiple imaging modalities are often required to fully characterize this disease.

The combined use of nuclear scintigraphy and MRI offers complementary information and may allow the clinical significance of multiple lesions to be determined. The most common distribution of palmar/plantar IRU is medial or biaxial in the front limb and lateral in the hind limb.[26] MRI offers anatomic detail that is not provided with nuclear scintigraphy. Current scintigraphic techniques may not be able to differentiate condylar and parasagittal uptake well. This limitation may be a consequence of inadequate image resolution or a similar subchondral bone response to both palmar condyle osteochondral disease or fracture and parasagittal fracture. Additional scintigraphic views, such as flexed dorsal views, may better differentiate parasagittal from condylar IRU (**Fig. 5**). Scintigraphy of horses that are lame or performing poorly does not seem to be an effective screening technique for condylar fractures. Bone fatigue associated with condylar fracture may develop rapidly and be present in sound horses. This process can result in fractures before an osteoblastic response that is evident scintigraphically.[26]

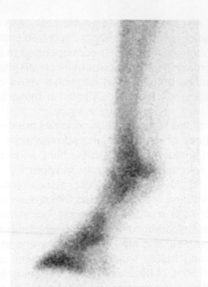

Fig. 4. Bone scan of the metacarpophalangeal joint showing adaptive changes of the palmarodistal McIII and palmaroproximal P1 associated with stress remodeling that showed no abnormalities radiographically.

Osteoarthritis of the Metacarpophalangeal and Metatarsophalangeal Joints

In Thoroughbred racehorses with lameness localized to the fetlock joint, metacarpophalangeal joint osteoarthritis is the most frequently diagnosed abnormality on subsequent MRI examination after inconclusive radiographic and ultrasonographic examinations.[16] Radiographic evidence of periarticular osteophytosis and osseous remodeling secondary to chronic synovitis occurs late in disease, and MRI seems to be the most comprehensive modality for assessing osteoarthritis of the fetlock.[19] The superior contrast resolution of MRI outperforms the higher spatial resolution of CT for recognizing degenerative disease. Because of the tomographic nature of those

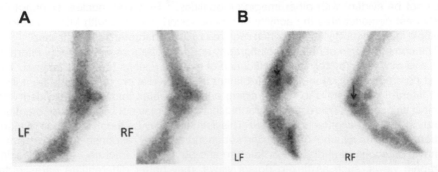

Fig. 5. (*A*) Bone scan in a weight-bearing position. Mild diffuse IRU of both metacarpophalangeal joints is seen, which is worse on the left compared with the right. (*B*) Bone scan of both metacarpophalangeal joints in flexion. Compared with the weight-bearing position, a focal IRU is not evident at the palmarodistal aspect of the distal McIII condyles (*arrows*). This finding corresponded to subchondral sclerosis from adaptive remodeling found in the MRI examination.

modalities, CT and MRI have increased sensitivity for detecting osteophytes compared with radiography.[19] Cartilage injury and degeneration result in wear lines or erosions that can be identified with high-field MRI as a focal accumulation of hyperintense joint fluid in cartilage defects on PD and STIR images.[17] Damage to or degeneration of articular cartilage can be inferred from detection of pathologic features in the subchondral bone, particularly with DR or MRI (1.0T).[18] However, DR underestimates the degree of subchondral sclerosis[19] and MRI generally underestimates the size and extent of cartilage loss compared with arthroscopy in accessible regions of the joint.[17]

Although MRI is accepted as the most suitable modality for cartilage imaging, accurate identification of cartilage lesions using MRI remains difficult in the metacarpophalangeal and metatarsophalangeal joints because of the thin cartilage and curved articular surfaces resulting in susceptibility to partial-volume averaging.[27,28] Sequences such as the T1-weighted spoiled gradient recalled acquisition at steady state (SPGR) with and without fat suppression (FS) were used in one study to examine the cartilage of the fetlock joint in cadaveric limbs.[28] That study showed that the SPGR and SPGR FS sequences best delineate the subchondral bone and cartilage in the carpus compared with a gradient echo (GRE) sequence.[28] Furthermore, the SPGR or SPGR FS sequences can be used to measure the cartilage thickness, because they both compare well to actual cartilage thickness histopathologically. Cartilage erosions can be detected consistently with moderate sensitivity and excellent specificity, and thickness can also be measured accurately using those image sequences. Another study examined experimentally induced osteochondral defects in the metacarpophalangeal joints of cadaver limbs to compare the effect of sequence selection and field strength on detection of articular cartilage defects. That study found that the number of cartilage lesions in the metacarpophalangeal joint identified using a low-field system was lower than with a high-field system. Furthermore, on both high- and low-field systems, turbo and fast spin echo sequences more accurately represented the size and shape of articular cartilage lesions compared with the GRE sequences.[29] This finding may be explained by the fact that in fat-suppressed PD, T2 turbo spin echo, and T2 fast spin echo sequences, articular cartilage has a low to intermediate signal, whereas chondral defects and fluid have a high signal, with more conspicuous contrast between the lower signal of cartilage and the higher signal of cartilage defects that are filled with high signal fluid. Detecting small lower-signal lesions in a background of high-signal surrounding cartilage may be difficult, and the conspicuity of the low-signal lesions may be further decreased by partial volume averaging with the high-signal surrounding intact cartilage.[29] Additionally, the contrast between the articular cartilage and the adjacent synovial fluid on GRE sequences tends to be low, particularly in fat-suppressed images.[29]

Osteophytes associated with osteoarthritis of the fetlock are generally identified radiographically and with MRI as contour changes of the proximal and distal articular margins of the sesamoid bones and periarticular margins of the P1.[17] T1-GRE and SPGR sequences detect periarticular osteophytes at a similar rate compared with CT. Smaller osteophytes are more accurately diagnosed with CT, because susceptibility artifacts that occur with GRE pulse sequences can result in overestimation of their size.[19] However, when evaluating the metacarpophalangeal/metatarsophalangeal joint for osteoarthritis, one must remember that the relationship between the presence of osteophytes and cartilage remains unclear.

Osteochondral fragments (chip fractures) of the proximodorsal aspect of the P1 are common in Thoroughbred racehorses. The fragments are usually medial but can be biaxial and bilateral. They are typically found in the fetlock at the dorsoproximal margin of the P1 or dorsal sagittal ridge of McIII. One study showed poor agreement with actual abnormality for detecting proximal P1 osteochondral fractures and condylar small cracks and lucencies using either radiography or CT. Radiography can be used to evaluate the dorsal rim of P1, enhancing the ability to detect fragments near the site of origin. CT allows examination of only the plane that the slice samples, and displacement of small fragments away from the dorsal rim could result in the fragment not being represented in an appropriate slice on the CT images. Palmar/plantar proximal P1 fragments are often small (<0.5 mm) and originate from the concave proximal rim of P1. The shape of the proximal P1 and the size of the fragments make them difficult to detect with either radiography or CT. Radiography was found to be best suited for detecting dorsal P1 fragments compared with CT, but neither radiography nor CT was adequate for detecting palmar/plantar fragments (60% missed).[24] However, this study did not include sagittal reconstructions, which would allow identification of these fragments, and the results of this study should be interpreted in light of this information.

The visibility of osteochondral fragments on MRI as opposed to radiographs depends on the fragment location and adjacent tissues. Summation effects in radiography can allow osteochondral fragments to be more readily apparent than on MRI, in which a fragment could be divided over 2 contiguous slices, decreasing its visibility. Osteochondral fragments have focal hypointensity or mixed signal intensity on MR images and are separated from the parent bone. An osseous fragment can be difficult to identify on an MR study. This difficulty arises because the osteochondral fragment has low signal intensity, similar to many adjacent structures, such as end-on blood vessels, tendon or ligament insertion sites, and adjacent joint capsule or synovial proliferation. Conversely, MRI eliminates superimposition and can allow for detection of osseous fragments not visualized radiographically. Neither radiography nor MRI offers a complete evaluation of osteoarthritis, and the most comprehensive evaluation would likely involve a combination of both techniques.[17]

Proximal Sesamoid Bone Injury

Injury of the proximal sesamoid bones of the metacarpophalangeal and metatarsophalangeal joints is usually not an isolated finding. Proximal sesamoid bone fractures have been well described and can be associated with catastrophic and noncatastrophic injury, depending on their severity. Although these injuries are readily diagnosed radiographically, CT may aid in presurgical planning of complex fractures. Abnormal MR signal in the proximal sesamoid bones, such as STIR hyperintensity, can be seen due to bone edema-like lesions, or as hypointense signal on PD, T1-weighted, and T2-weighted images due to osteosclerosis.[17] Small, osseous cyst-like lesions at the base of the proximal sesamoid bones can be seen associated with damage to the attachment of the straight distal sesamoidean ligament[17] or oblique distal sesamoidean ligaments. Osteolytic lesions at the axial margin of a sesamoid bone can also be associated with intersesamoidean desmitis, sesamoiditis, and adaptive remodeling. Bone scintigraphy shows IRU of the affected sesamoids in these cases. However, Thoroughbred racehorses generally have adaptive changes in the proximal sesamoids that are not biaxially symmetric and must be distinguished from pathologic change (**Fig. 6**).

Soft Tissue Injury of the Metacarpophalangeal/Metatarsophalangeal Joints

Ultrasonography of the palmar/plantar aspect of the fetlock is indicated for assessing distension of the digital sheath, presence of soft tissue thickening, concurrent distal metacarpal/metatarsal tendinopathy, suspensory branch injuries, or metacarpophalangeal/metatarsophalangeal arthropathy.[30] Ligaments of the metacarpophalangeal/metatarsophalangeal regions that should be assessed in the presence of soft tissue swelling include the suspensory ligament, straight distal sesamoidean ligament

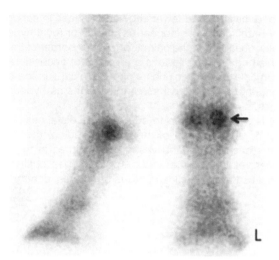

Fig. 6. Bone scan of the left metatarsophalangeal joint showing focal IRU of the lateral proximal sesamoid bone (*arrow*). No abnormalities were found on ultrasound, radiography, or MRI of the region, and the changes were assessed as adaptive remodeling seen frequently in that bone in Thoroughbred racehorses.

(SDSL), oblique distal sesamoidean ligament (ODSL), proximal aspect of the collateral sesamoidean ligaments, and the collateral ligaments.[31,32] Additional indications include a positive distal metacarpal/metatarsal nerve block, abnormal radiographic findings of the proximal sesamoid bones, and increased radiopharmaceutical uptake over the palmar/plantar fetlock area on nuclear scintigraphy.[30]

Although suspensory branch injury is commonly diagnosed with ultrasound, it has been shown to be best identified with MRI (**Fig. 7**).[17] In one study, enlargement of the branches could only be detected sonographically in approximately half of the

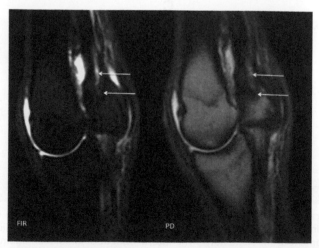

Fig. 7. MRI STIR (*left*) and proton density (*right*) images of the lateral suspensory branch showing focal hyperintensity of the ligament, with extension of the signal change into the sesamoid bone (*arrows*). Suspensory branch desmitis was diagnosed and was not evident on the ultrasound examination.

horses with MR abnormalities, and fewer showed changes in echogenicity. MR findings in suspensory branch desmitis appear as diffuse or focal hyperintensity on PD, T2, and STIR images, usually near the palmar or plantar border of the affected branch, which is usually enlarged.[17] These lesions are often not accessible arthroscopically. MR imaging is often able to show injuries along the axial surface of the suspensory branches, extending into the proximal sesamoid bones as hyperintense signals on PD and STIR images.[33]

Ultrasonography is commonly used to evaluate the distal sesamoidean ligaments (**Fig. 8**). However, the conformation of the pastern region, the multiple soft tissue structures of various orientations, and vascular structures in this region can make production and interpretation of the sonographic images challenging. MRI better delineates the complex anatomy of ligamentous structures, accurately characterizing

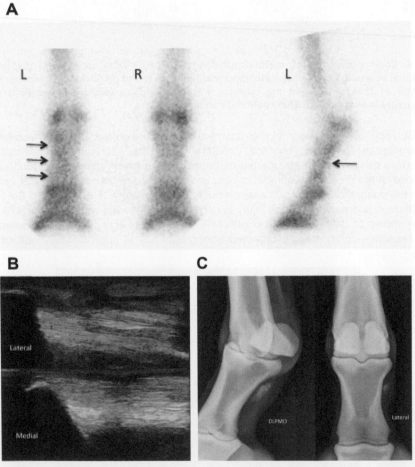

Fig. 8. (*A*) Focal IRU of the palmarolateral aspect of the P1 (*arrows*) of the left limb and normal right limb. (*B*) Sagittal ultrasound images of the lateral and medial oblique distal sesamoidean ligament of the same horse. The lateral oblique sesamoidean ligament has a disrupted fiber pattern with linear hypoechoic defects. (*C*) Radiographic images of the same horse showing dystrophic mineralization at the site of the lateral oblique distal sesamoidean ligament representing chronic desmitis from tearing. *Abbreviations:* DLPMO, dorsolateral palmaromedial oblique

fat and facial planes from regions of ligament fibers. These multiple tissue types complicate ultrasound examination and create a mixed signal pattern on MRI. Injuries to the ODSL result in increased size of the ligament and increased MRI signal intensity. The increased signal intensity can be diffuse or focal and can be located centrally or peripherally within the ligament. The SDSL seems to be less susceptible to injury than the ODSL, but SDSL injury does occur.[14] Ultrasonographic correlation to lesions in the distal sesamoidean ligaments diagnosed with MRI has shown that subtle lesions could be detected retrospectively.[17] Injuries can occur anywhere throughout the SDSL and often involve diffuse areas of intermediate signal intensity, although core lesions can occur.[33] The SDSL shows variable signal intensity as it blends distally with the fibro-cartilaginous middle scutum, which should be distinguished from increased signal caused by injury at this location. MR signal characteristics of distal sesamoidean ligament desmitis are focal or generalized hyperintensity on PD, T2-weighted, and STIR images. Small core lesions with a focal signal increase can also be observed.[17] Lesions have been identified at or near the origin of the SDSL and ODSL and have been reported to be less common at the insertion.[17]

The normal intersesamoidean ligament has mixed signal intensity on T2 and PD images, with some signal variation on STIR images. Intersesamoidean ligament desmitis appears as hyperintensity on T2, PD, and STIR images (**Fig. 9**). An abnormal contour can be identified at the axial margin of the proximal sesamoid bone on MRI, resulting from bone resorption associated with intersesamoidean ligament desmitis. This contour change can also often be identified radiographically. Because of multiple fiber orientations within the ligament, intersesamoidean ligament desmitis can be difficult to diagnose sonographically.

CARPAL LAMENESS

The carpus is a frequent site of lameness, but usually not involved in catastrophic injuries. Radiography is the most common modality for examining the carpus, because carpal osteochondral fragments (chips) and slab fractures are diagnosed adequately in most instances. However, small fragments may be difficult to detect. Although mild pathologic change is not uncommon, the radial and third carpal bones can be significant sites of disease. The radial facet of the C3 has been hypothesized to undergo extreme bone formation, to the point that the subchondral bone becomes ischemic and necrotic, resulting in collapse of the overlying cartilage.[2] Nonadaptive remodeling of the third and radial carpal bones is common in Thoroughbred racehorses, and pain originating from the carpus, carpal sheath, and proximal metacarpal region can be difficult to differentiate clinically.

C3 Disease

Sclerosis of C3 is best seen on skyline radiographic projections of the distal row of carpal bones as a zone of opacity accentuated at the radial facet. This condition can be a source of pain caused by nonadaptive remodeling. Bone scintigraphy is an excellent screening test for stress-related injury to the carpus and can help in early diagnosis of C3 stress remodeling (**Fig. 10**).

Recently, MRI has been used to assess stress remodeling of this area. MRI can detect thickening of the subchondral bone plate seen histologically but not radiographically,[34] because thin MR imaging slices can be oriented through areas of specific interest, in this case directly under the proximal articular surface of the radial facet of C3, where bone remodeling is expected to occur. This result cannot be achieved with conventional radiography, which is not as sensitive as MR imaging in

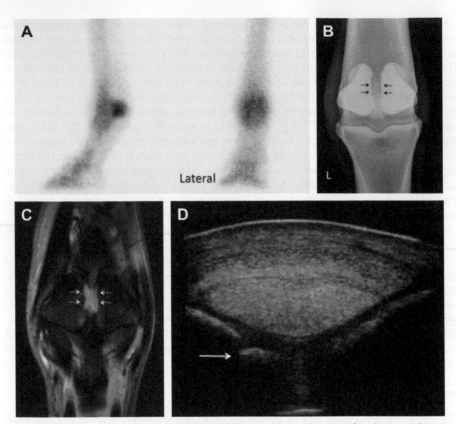

Fig. 9. (*A*) Bone scan of the left metatarsophalangeal joint showing focal IRU at the sesamoid bones but appearing diffuse on the dorsoplantar image. (*B*) Dorsoplantar radiographs of the same horse showing focal, mild concavity of the medial border of both proximal sesamoid bones (*arrows*). (*C*) STIR MRI dorsal plane MRI image of the same horse showing diffuse hyperintensity of the intersesamoidean ligament from desmitis. (*D*) Ultrasound image of the same horse at the plantar aspect of the metatarsophalangeal joint showing a focal defect in the medial proximal sesamoid bone at its medial aspect. No abnormalities of the ligament itself could be appreciated. This surface of the sesamoid can have focal depressions as part of the normal anatomy, and this appearance should be interpreted with caution.

detecting early bone changes.[34] Whether MR imaging or CT can detect stress fractures or microfractures in the C3, and which is more sensitive and specific as part of the continuum of stress-induced injury, are not yet known.

Many racehorses also have radiographic evidence of adaptive or degenerative change associated with the distal carpus, which may not be of primary clinical relevance and should be distinguished from proximal suspensory ligament (PSL) disease. Although scintigraphic evaluation may help differentiate carpal pain from proximal metacarpal pain, active adaptive remodeling occurs in racing and training Thoroughbreds, resulting in IRU, and can be difficult to distinguish from bone injury.[35]

Subcarpal/Third Metacarpal Disease

Ultrasonography is commonly used to identify PSL disease, but the normal and diseased ligament show considerable variation.[7] The PSL of the forelimb has

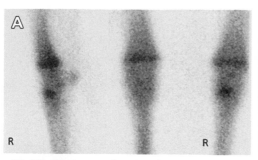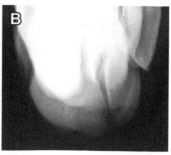

Fig. 10. (A). Bone scan showing focal IRU of the C3. The distal radial physis is increased because of the young age of the horse. (B). Extensive sclerosis of the C3 in the same horse at the radial facet, which corresponds to the IRU on the bone scan and the source of pain in this horse.

a heterogeneous ultrasonographic appearance. Variation in the size of the ligament and the amount of muscular and adipose tissue is common. As a result, hypoechoic areas within the ligament caused by normal anatomy can also be identified in sound horses and must be differentiated from hypoechoic areas caused by ligamentous damage. Osseous injury of the proximal palmar aspect of McIII can also be seen in horses without obvious tearing of the PSL. When these cases have negative radiographic findings, scintigraphy or MRI is required to diagnose osseous damage. Incomplete and avulsion fractures of the palmar cortex of proximal McIII, bone resorption at the suspensory ligament attachment, and bone contusions lead to intense IRU (Fig. 11).

MRI offers advantages over radiography and ultrasonography when investigating suspected subcarpal lameness.[32,36] MR findings associated with suspensory desmitis include thickening of the PSL, adhesions between the PSL and the adjacent metacarpal/metatarsal bones, diffuse fiber abnormality, and core lesions.[33] Adhesions of the PSL to the metacarpal or metatarsal bones result in an area of abnormal tissue traversing the high signal intensity connective tissue between the PSL and McIII. Core lesions and diffuse fiber injury result in increased signal intensity within the PSL caused by fluid and increased cellularity within the ligament after trauma.

Horses with lameness localized to the carpus or subcarpal region that have negative ultrasonographic and radiographic findings can show signal abnormality within the palmaroproximal aspect of McIII, comprising hypointensity on T1-weighted GRE images corresponding with hyperintensity on T2-weighted fast spin echo and STIR images.[6] These signal patterns indicate the presence of fluid, and most likely represent proximal McIII stress reactions, and these osseous changes have been hypothesized to be the primary source of pain in absence of injury to the ligament.[6] In the palmar cortical bone of McIII, the lesion is thought to be a radiographically silent cortical stress fracture that can present as an endosteal reaction 3 to 10 months later radiographically.[6]

DORSAL METACARPAL DISEASE

Dorsal metacarpal disease (bucked shins) results from microfractures in the dorsal cortex caused by high-speed exercise. Large surface strains measured in vivo at high speeds on the dorsolateral aspect of McIII in young Thoroughbred racehorses in training contrasts dramatically with the smaller strains measured in adults that

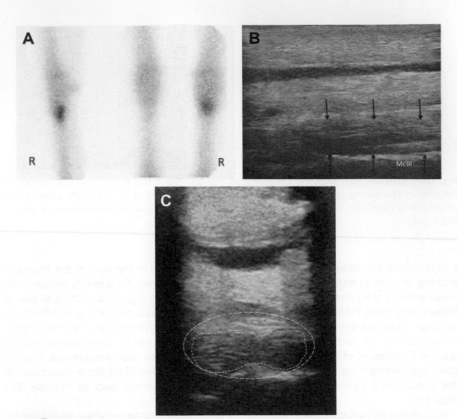

Fig. 11. (A) Bone scan showing focal IRU at the palmaroproximal aspect of the McIII bone in the region of the origin of the suspensory ligament. This appearance can be seen with proximal suspensory desmitis and avulsion, or incomplete fracture of the palmar cortex of MCIII and contusion in this region. (B) Dorsopalmar radiograph showing a radiolucent region bordered by sclerosis in the proximal third metacarpus (*arrows*). (C) Sagittal ultrasound image of the proximal suspensory ligament of the same horse showing an irregular bony contour and focal hypoechoic zone with fiber disruption.

have raced successfully.[37] Both tensile and compressive strain occur at dorsal McIII during exercise. Bone that adapts to tensile strain (at slow gaits) may not be able to resist compressive strains (high speed) in the same location. Strain, under a given load, relates to the inertial properties of the bone, which increase with age. Bone strain during high-speed exercise has been shown to decrease in older horses.[37] However, training regimens can outpace this adaptive response, and young horses have increased strain at dorsal McIII after several months of training.[37] The high incidence of bucked shins in Thoroughbred racehorses suggests that loading to produce peak strains and concomitant adaptive remodeling does not always occur in many horses in training programs.

Radiographically, horses with dorsal cortical stress remodeling can show a range of severity from dorsal periosteal and endosteal thickening to dorsal cortical fractures and sequestrum formation (**Fig. 12**). Scintigraphy is useful for detecting stress fractures and shows focal regions of IRU (**Fig. 13**). The use of MRI and CT has not been reported for the examination of dorsal cortical disease, and radiography is generally considered to be adequate.

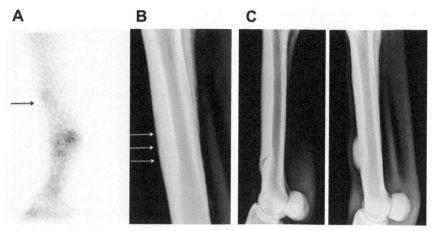

Fig. 12. (*A*) Focal IRU (*arrow*) at the dorsal mid-third metacarpus. (*B*) Lateral radiograph of the same horse showing mild thickening of the dorsal cortex of McIII and mild heterogeneity of the cortical opacity. These findings represent adaptive remodeling of the dorsal metacarpus (*arrows*). (*C*) Two different Thoroughbred racehorses with cortical stress fractures. The lateral radiograph on the left shows a typical saucer fracture with callus formation, whereas the image on the right is from a horse with a chronic injury and extensive callus formation, showing how the disease can progress if left untreated.

TIBIAL STRESS REMODELING AND FRACTURES

Tibial stress fractures are a common cause of acute, unilateral hind limb lameness in thoroughbred racehorses. These fractures are usually unilateral, but bilateral fractures can cause hind limb lameness. Scintigraphy is the preferred imaging modality for diagnosis, and its use has led to the early detection of stress fractures.[38] Fewer than 50% of horses diagnosed with tibial stress fractures using scintigraphy have radiographically apparent fractures, even on follow-up examination 2 weeks later.[7] Diagnosis of tibial stress fractures relies of radiographic evidence of endosteal, periosteal, and cortical changes, and these radiographic abnormalities lag behind IRU associated with acute tibial stress fractures.

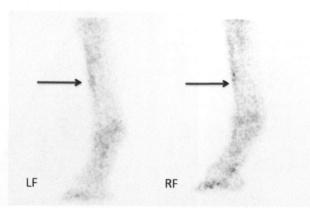

Fig. 13. Lateral bone scans of both front metacarpal regions showing a linear pattern of IRU (*arrows*) along the dorsal border of McIII representing adaptive remodeling. No radiographic changes were evident.

Three predilection sites have been described: the proximolateral cortex, the caudal cortex of the mid-shaft, and the caudal cortex of the distal tibia (**Fig. 14**). A 0 to 4 scale of scintigraphic and radiographic grading has been recommended[38]:

0: normal
1: small, ill-defined area of mild IRU
2: IRU greater than grade 1 but without well-marginated borders
3: well-marginated focal IRU
4: well-marginated IRU extending over a larger area

Radiographic grading has been described on a 0 to 3 scale:

0: normal
1: subtle diffuse intramedullary sclerosis
2: moderate endosteal and/or periosteal proliferation
3: marked endosteal and/or periosteal callus and possible presence of cortical linear lucency suggestive of a fracture

Using this grading system, a significant association between scintigraphic and radiographic grades can be demonstrated in Thoroughbred racehorses.[38] Proximal lesions have significantly higher grades than at other sites both scintigraphically and radiographically, and mid-diaphyseal lesions have the lowest grades.[38] Furthermore, proximal and distal IRU is more likely to be bilateral than mid-diaphyseal lesions.[38] However, no significant associations were found between scintigraphic grade and radiographic grade or radiographic grade and degree of lameness, nor was any significant association seen between scintigraphic grade and degree of lameness. Therefore, the usefulness of a grading system for determining prognosis or developing a therapeutic plan of rest versus controlled exercise is unclear and will require larger longitudinal studies.

HUMERAL STRESS FRACTURES

Humeral stress fractures also occur in Thoroughbred racehorses and have bone scan and radiographic findings similar to tibial stress fractures. Catastrophic humeral

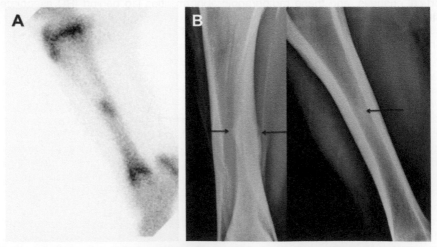

Fig. 14. (*A*) Bone scan showing IRU at the caudal aspect of the mid-tibial diaphysis. (*B*) Orthogonal radiographs of the same tibia showing focal sclerosis, and endosteal and periosteal new bone formation (*arrows*) representing a stress fracture.

fractures are typically seen in Thoroughbred racehorses during training compared with racing.[37] Evidence of stress remodeling as an underlying cause of catastrophic fractures has also been observed in association with fractures of the McIII bone, humerus, scapula, carpal cuboidal bones, and the pelvis or vertebrae.[3]

TENDONITIS AND DESMITIS
Superficial Digital Flexor Tendonitis

Superficial digital flexor tendonitis is a major source of injury in Thoroughbred racehorses. Damage to the superficial digital flexor tendon (SDFT) can occur anywhere along the metacarpus or metatarsus, but tends to be more common in the mid-metacarpal region and usually occurs mainly in the front limb of Thoroughbred racehorses.[39] "Low bows" in the distal metacarpus are the next most common location in Thoroughbred racehorses. Lesions can be seen as an increase in size, tearing, and disruption of fiber pattern and/or discrete core lesions. Lesions of the SDFT are particularly common in horses that work at speed. Even small tears can cause lameness and require time to recover before return to training. Ultrasonography should be performed at the earliest instance after swelling or inflammation in the flexor tendons is identified. Ultrasonographic examination should always include cross-sectional area measurements and/or comparison to the opposite limb, because subtle enlargements of the SDFT will precede fiber tearing.

Although ultrasound remains a useful tool for diagnosing tendon lesions, MRI is capable of detecting subtle changes in tissue composition that are not detectable ultrasonographically. When viewed with MRI, normal tendons have low signal intensity, regardless of the sequence used to acquire the images. The connective tissue framework of tendons is more apparent on certain sequences. On MR images, the response to injury is seen as a change in size or shape, or an alteration of signal intensity. Like ultrasound, MRI detects enlargement and change in the tissue composition of the tendon or ligament.[33]

The appearance of a tendon lesion on MRI depends on the stage of healing. Acute tears that contain a great deal of hemorrhage and edema produce high signal intensity on STIR, T2-weighted, T1-weighted, and PD images. On STIR, T2, and PD images, core lesions with fiber disruption are visible as a focal area of high signal intensity representing the fluid and hypercellularity within the tendon. Hemorrhage within the tendon can produce high signals on T1-weighted images in the acute phase. In a study examining experimentally induced tendon injury and compared ultrasound and MRI images to histopathology from 2 to 16 weeks' postinjury, MRI signal intensity of lesions was greatest for T1-weighted images, intermediate for STIR images, and lowest for T2-weighted images at all instances.[40] Yet another study showed that equine tendon injuries can have a persistent increase in T1-weighted signal intensity for more than 6 months after the onset of injury, whereas the T2-weighted signal intensity decreased over time.[41] A decrease in proteoglycan content corresponds with the slow decrease in T2 signal intensities of the tendon lesions seen on MRI images over time.[40] Hemorrhage and inflammation are the likely causes of the increased T1-weighted signal in the acute phase, but why the T1-weighted signal remains increased chronically is unclear. For monitoring purposes, T2-weighted images may be more practical, because the lesion signal intensity decreases as the tendon heals, but the T1-weighted intensities persist indefinitely.[40] "Healed" tendon lesions have a variable appearance depending on tissue content. Both scarring and realigned tendon fibers can have high signal intensity on T1-weighted images.[40,41] However, in the early fibrogenesis stage of tendon healing, MR images can show mixed signal intensity, whereas ultrasonography can reveal the continued presence of a hypoechoic lesion in the same horse.[42]

In experimentally induced SDFT lesions, MRI and ultrasound have shown similar results for the cross-sectional area of the damaged tendon. At greater than 4 weeks' postinduction of tendonitis, however, ultrasound underestimated the cross-sectional size of lesions compared with MRI.[40]

Deep Digital Flexor Tendonitis

As with the SDFT, most imaging of the deep digital flexor tendon (DDFT) at the meta-carpal/metatarsal and pastern regions is performed sonographically. Tendon lesions in the fetlock region often occur at the level of the proximal third of the P1 and extend proximally to the level of the proximal sesamoid bones.[17] Few reports compare ultra-sound with MRI for examination of the DDFT in the fetlock region. Mild enlargement of the tendon identified sonographically can be associated with a region of signal change on MRI.[17] Much work has been done to describe DDFT lesions within the hoof capsule identified using MRI. This region is difficult to examine using ultrasound, and marked limitations exist in characterizing certain injuries. These limitations result from the presence of the hoof capsule and the orientation of the DDFT at this level in conjunc-tion with the probe position required to perform this examination. Deep digital flexor tendon injury can present as a variety of appearances on MR images, depending on the severity and extent of disease. Tendonitis can appear as small, focal areas of hyperintensity throughout the tendon, whereas more severe injury can have focal hyperintensity from core lesions or parasagittal split. Focal or diffuse enlargement accompanies most of these conditions. The sequence that best demonstrates the lesion depends on the lesion type and severity and the adjacent tissues.

SUMMARY

Orthopedic injuries in Thoroughbred racehorses are most commonly diagnosed with radiography, bone scintigraphy, and ultrasonography. Radiography and bone scintig-raphy allow the diagnosis of most osseous injuries, such as stress fractures and oste-oarthritis, and are widely available. Ultrasonography remains the most important modality for diagnosing tendon injuries of the distal extremities, but early work with MRI is showing that this modality has advantages for diagnosing proximal suspensory desmitis. MRI is now recognized for its important role in diagnosing subchondral disease that is radiographically silent. Adaptive and nonadaptive osseous changes in the subchondral bone and cortical bone are important sources of lameness in the Thoroughbred racehorse that relate to many circumstances, including training prac-tices, track conditions, and age. Future areas of study will need to focus on how imaging findings relate to prognosis and whether they can help accurately formulate therapeutic strategies in athletic horses.

REFERENCES

1. Kawcak CE, McIlwraith CW, Norrdin RW, et al. The role of subchondral bone in joint disease: a review. Equine Vet J 2001;33:120–6.
2. Pool RR, Meagher DM. Pathologic findings and pathogenesis of racetrack injuries. Vet Clin North Am Equine Pract 1990;6:1–30.
3. Stover SL. Epidemiology of thoroughbred racehorse injuries. Clin Tech Equine Pract 2003;2:312–22.

4. Whitton RC, Trope GD, Ghasem-Zadeh A, et al. Third metacarpal condylar fatigue fractures in equine athletes occur within previously modelled subchondral bone. Bone 2010;47:826–31.

5. Rubin CT, Lanyon LE. Kappa Delta Award paper. Osteoregulatory nature of mechanical stimuli: function as a determinant for adaptive remodeling in bone. J Orthop Res 1987;5:300–10.

6. Powell SE, Ramzan PH, Head MJ, et al. Standing magnetic resonance imaging detection of bone marrow oedema-type signal pattern associated with subcarpal pain in 8 racehorses: a prospective study. Equine Vet J 2010;42:10–7.

7. Arthur RM, Ross MW, Maloney PJ, et al. North American Thoroughbred. In: Ross MW, Dysone SJ, editors. Lameness in the Horse. St Louis (MO): Saunders; 2003. p. 868–78.

8. Archer DC, Boswell JC, Voute LC, et al. Skeletal scintigraphy in the horse: current indications and validity as a diagnostic test. Vet J 2007;173:31–44.

9. Young BD, Samii VF, Mattoon JS, et al. Subchondral bone density and cartilage degeneration patterns in osteoarthritic metacarpal condyles of horses. Am J Vet Res 2007;68:841–9.

10. Murray RC, Blunden TS, Schramme MC, et al. How does magnetic resonance imaging represent histologic findings in the equine digit? Vet Radiol Ultrasound 2006;47:17–31.

11. Perrin RA, Launois MT, Brogniez L, et al. The use of computed tomography to assist orthopaedic surgery in 86 horses (2002-1010). Equine Vet Educ 2011;23:306–13.

12. Zubrod CJ, Schneider RK, Tucker RL, et al. Use of magnetic resonance imaging for identifying subchondral bone damage in horses: 11 cases (1999-2003). J Am Vet Med Assoc 2004;224:411–8.

13. Sherlock CE, Mair TS, Ter Braake F. Osseous lesions in the metacarpo(tarso) phalangeal joint diagnosed using low-field magnetic resonance imaging in standing horses. Vet Radiol Ultrasound 2009;50:13–20.

14. Sampson SN, Schneider RK, Tucker RL, et al. Magnetic resonance imaging features of oblique and straight distal sesamoidean desmitis in 27 horses. Vet Radiol Ultrasound 2007;48:303–11.

15. Smith S, Dyson SJ, Murray RC. Magnetic resonance imaging of distal sesamoidean ligament injury. Vet Radiol Ultrasound 2008;49:516–28.

16. Dyson S, Murray RC. Magnetic resonance imaging of the equine fetlock. Clin Tech Equine Pract 2007;6:62–77.

17. Gonzalez LM, Schramme MC, Robertson ID, et al. MRI features of metacarpo (tarso)phalangeal region lameness in 40 horses. Vet Radiol Ultrasound 2010; 51:404–14.

18. O'Brien T, Baker TA, Brounts SH, et al. Detection of articular pathology of the distal aspect of the third metacarpal bone in thoroughbred racehorses: comparison of radiography, computed tomography and magnetic resonance imaging. Vet Surg 2011;40:942–51.

19. Olive J, D'Anjou MA, Alexander K, et al. Comparison of magnetic resonance imaging, computed tomography, and radiography for assessment of noncartilaginous changes in equine metacarpophalangeal osteoarthritis. Vet Radiol Ultrasound 2010;51:267–79.

20. Riggs CM, Whitehouse GH, Boyde A. Structural variation of the distal condyles of the third metacarpal and third metatarsal bones in the horse. Equine Vet J 1999; 31:130–9.

21. Beccati F, Pepe M, Di Meo A, et al. Radiographic evaluation of changes in the proximal phalanx of Thoroughbreds in race training. Am J Vet Res 2011;72:1482–8.

22. Parkin TD. Epidemiology of racetrack injuries in racehorses. Vet Clin North Am Equine Pract 2008;24:1–19.
23. Ramzan PH, Powell SE. Clinical and imaging features of suspected prodromal fracture of the proximal phalanx in three Thoroughbred racehorses. Equine Vet J 2010;42:164–9.
24. Morgan JW, Santschi EM, Zekas LJ, et al. Comparison of radiography and computed tomography to evaluate metacarpo/metatarsophalangeal joint pathology of paired limbs of thoroughbred racehorses with severe condylar fracture. Vet Surg 2006;35:611–7.
25. Barr ED, Pinchbeck GL, Clegg PD, et al. Post mortem evaluation of palmar osteochondral disease (traumatic osteochondrosis) of the metacarpo/metatarsophalangeal joint in Thoroughbred racehorses. Equine Vet J 2009;41:366–71.
26. Trope GD, Anderson GA, Whitton RC. Patterns of scintigraphic uptake in the fetlock joint of Thoroughbred racehorses and the effect of increased radiopharmaceutical uptake in the distal metacarpal/tarsal condyle on performance. Equine Vet J 2011;43(5):509–15.
27. Murray RC, Branch MV, Tranquille C, et al. Validation of magnetic resonance imaging for measurement of equine articular cartilage and subchondral bone thickness. Am J Vet Res 2005;66:1999–2005.
28. Olive J, D'Anjou MA, Girard C, et al. Fat-suppressed spoiled gradient-recalled imaging of equine metacarpophalangeal articular cartilage. Vet Radiol Ultrasound 2010;51:107–15.
29. Werpy NM, Ho CP, Pease AP, et al. The effect of sequence selection and field strength on detection of osteochondral defects in the metacarpophalangeal joint. Vet Radiol Ultrasound 2011;52:154–60.
30. Seignour M, Coudry V, Norris R, et al. Ultrasonographic examination of the palmar/plantar aspect of the fetlock in the horse: technique and normal images. Equine Vet Educ 2012;24:19–29.
31. Zubrod CJ, Farnsworth KD, Tucker RL, et al. Injury of the collateral ligaments of the distal interphalangeal joint diagnosed by magnetic resonance. Vet Radiol Ultrasound 2005;46:11–6.
32. Zubrod CJ, Schneider RK, Tucker RL. Use of magnetic resonance imaging identify suspensory desmitis and adhesions between exostoses of the second metacarpal bone and the suspensory ligament in four horses. J Am Vet Med Assoc 2004;224:1815–20.
33. Zubrod CJ, Barrett MF. Magnetic resonance imaging of tendon and ligament injuries. Clin Tech Equine Pract 2007;6:217–29.
34. Anastasioiu A, Skioldebrand E, Ekman S, et al. Ex vivo magnetic resonance imaging of the distal row of equine carpal bones: assessment of bone sclerosis and cartilage damage. Vet Radiol Ultrasound 2003;44:501–12.
35. Dyson SJ, Weekes JS, Murray RC. Scintigraphic evaluation of the proximal metacarpal and metatarsal regions of horses with proximal suspensory desmitis. Vet Radiol Ultrasound 2007;48:78–85.
36. Bischofberger AS, Konar M, Ohlerth S, et al. Magnetic resonance imaging, ultrasonography and histology of the suspensory ligament origin: a comparative study of normal anatomy of warmblood horses. Equine Vet J 2006;38:508–16.
37. Nunamaker DM. The bucked shin complex. In: Ross MW, Dyson SJ, editors. Lameness in the Horse. St Louis (MO): Saunders; 2003. p. 847–54.
38. Ramzan PH, Newton JR, Shepherd MC, et al. The application of a scintigraphic grading system to equine tibial stress fractures: 42 cases. Equine Vet J 2003;35:382–8.

39. Gillis CL, Meagher DM, Pool RR, et al. Ultrasonographically detected changes in equine superficial digital flexor tendons during the first months of race training. Am J Vet Res 1993;54:1797–802.
40. Karlin WM, Stewart AA, Durgam SS, et al. Evaluation of experimentally induced injury to the superficial digital flexor tendon in horses by use of low-field magnetic resonance imaging and ultrasonography. Am J Vet Res 2011;72:791–8.
41. Kasashima Y, Kuwano A, Katayama Y, et al. Magnetic resonance imaging application to live horse for diagnosis of tendinitis. J Vet Med Sci 2002;64:577–82.
42. Crass JR, Genovese RI, Render JA, et al. Magnetic resonance, ultrasound and histopathologic correlation of acute and healing equine tendon injuries. Vet Radiol Ultrasound 1992;33:206–16.

Advances in Equine Computed Tomography and Use of Contrast Media

Sarah M. Puchalski, DVM

KEYWORDS

- Computed tomography • Contrast enhanced computed tomography
- Contrast media

KEY POINTS

- Advances in equine computed tomography have been made as a result of improvements in software and hardware and an increasing body of knowledge.
- Contrast media can be administered intravascularly or intrathecally.
- Contrast media is useful to differentiate between tissues of similar density.
- Equine computed tomography can be used for many different clinical conditions, including lameness diagnosis, fracture identification and characterization, preoperative planning, and characterization of skull diseases.

INTRODUCTION

Of all specialties in health sciences, the digital age has impacted diagnostic imaging most significantly. Descriptively named, computed tomography (CT), previously known as computed axial tomography, is only possible because of modern computing technology. As a result of advances in computing technology, the practical clinical applications of CT have developed at a vigorous pace.

The clinical use of CT scanning in equine practice, like magnetic resonance (MR) imaging, is possible because of the ingenuity in adaptation of human centric technologies, advances in hardware and software, and an ever increasing body of knowledge specific to the technique and the species. CT scanning uses x-ray attenuation as the fundamental premise for image formation. Therefore, this technology is best suited to the evaluation of anatomy with varied inherent tissue density such as the osseous skeleton or the equine skull. Currently, CT scanners are most frequently used for the identification and characterization of musculoskeletal injuries in lameness diagnosis, the characterization of sinonasal, skull and dental disease, and trauma

Department of Surgical and Radiological Sciences, School of Veterinary Medicine, University of California, One Shields Avenue, Davis, Davis CA 95616, USA
E-mail address: smpuchalski@ucdavis.edu

Vet Clin Equine 28 (2012) 563–581
http://dx.doi.org/10.1016/j.cveq.2012.08.002
0749-0739/12/$ – see front matter © 2012 Elsevier Inc. All rights reserved.

particularly pertaining to fracture and surgical management, and other equine veterinary clinical conditions.

The strengths of CT are that it is a rapid, high spatial resolution, cross-sectional imaging modality that produces detailed, relatively user-friendly images. A weakness of the modality results from the technological limitation that tissues of similar density, such as synovial fluid and cartilage, are difficult to differentiate. This weakness is partially obviated by the use of contrast media in a variety of applications including contrast-enhanced CT (CE-CT), CT angiography, and CT arthrography. The goals of this report are to provide an overview of advances in CT scanning, addressing hardware and software advances and the use of contrast media, and to summarize recent advances in the field.

Hardware

- Helical and multislice CT technologies greatly increase CT scan speed.
- Table design is critical for equine scanning.
- Multislice CT technology allows for very thin slices.

Veterinary diagnostic imaging depends on research and development by human health care vendors and subsequent modification of the technology; CT is no exception. The scanner and the patient table are necessary hardware components for the practical use of CT in horses. Great advances in scanner technology have been made globally during the years, but the onus remains on veterinary-specific contractors for the development of equine CT tables.

All CT scans are produced by some variation of the same basic format: the anatomic region of interest is passed through the center of a circular gantry housing an x-ray generator and a detector apparatus.[1] This can be achieved by table motion or motion of the gantry, and both types of systems are in use in veterinary medicine. To obtain high-quality images, precision in table or gantry translation is required. The most common configuration is a stationary gantry with a 70- to 80-cm-diameter opening and an equine-suitable table married to the manufacturer's human couch, thus using the precision movement built into the CT scanner. Alternative options exist whereby the CT gantry moves around the stationary patient. In this arrangement, the CT scanners have been developed for use as an intraoperative aid or in the emergency department of human hospitals and are frequently furnished with smaller (30- to 35-cm)-diameter gantry openings than the stationary scanners.

Major advances in CT scanning have been achieved through hardware developments at the level of the gantry, greatly increasing scanning speed. These include helical scanning technology and the integration of multirow detectors.[1] Regardless of the methodology used to generate motion, most modern scanners use helical scanning technology. This advance allows for continuous circular motion of the x-ray generator and its associated detectors during relative patient translation through the gantry center. It is this advancement, in addition to the development of multirow detectors, that has provided the famously touted rapidity with which CT is credited. In a single-row detector scanner, the volume of tissue that could be scanned during one revolution of the gantry was determined by the slice thickness chosen at scan set-up: one slice or 1 to 10 mm of tissue per revolution. Multirow detectors allow for the acquisition of many images (as many images as detector rows) from a larger volume of tissue simultaneously.

In addition to greater speed, multirow or multislice CT scanners offer greater flexibility in image-acquisition parameters. Using this technology, several advantages can be realized. Very thin (<1 mm) slices and overlapping tissue slices can be obtained, the former allowing for increased resolution and the latter providing better material for manipulation with modern software such as multiplanar reformatting tools and 3-dimensional (3D) reconstructions.

The patient table is a critical hardware item. As stated previously, it is vital to have a very high degree of temporal and spatial precision in patient motion so that the anatomy is accurately represented in the acquired images. Table configuration will have a large influence on the anatomy that can be scanned. Newer table design, accommodating the hindquarters, has allowed for routine scanning of equine stifles (**Fig. 1**). Flexibility in patient positioning is important. The table design should be able to accommodate left, right, and dorsal recumbency and be able to include fore-limbs or hindlimbs within the gantry. These factors render table design technically challenging and the equine veterinary market is relatively small; subsequently, there are a limited number of equine table manufacturers. More recently, CT scanning of the equine skull has been achieved by standing a sedated horse on a hovercraft-design table (**Fig. 2**). The late Alastair Nelson of the United Kingdom conceptualized this major advancement and CT manufacturers have since adopted the technology.

Software

- Processing is achieved through software advances and can improve image quality or image utility.
- Postprocessing allows for manipulation of the images after they are acquired, including:
  - Window and level (brightness and contrast) control
  - Multiplanar reformatting or reslicing the images in planes other than the plane of acquisition
  - Three-dimensional models
- CT scans should be evaluated using a window width and level appropriate to the tissue of interest.

Routine evaluation of CT scans relies and incorporates many important software advances, which occur at the level of acquisition and image display.[1,2] The net result of these advances is to produce images that increase this technology's clinical utility and diagnostic accuracy. These advances, when applied to surgical planning or inter-vention, in turn reduce surgical time.

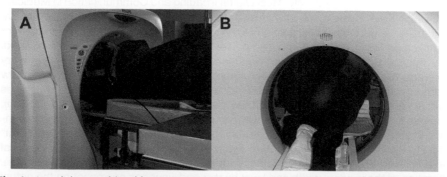

Fig. 1. An adult warmblood horse is positioned in a CT scanner to scan the left stifle at de Lingehoeve Diergeneeskunde, Lienden, the Netherlands. In A, the horse is seen from the table side of the gantry. In B, the limb is extended through the gantry for optimal posi-tioning of the hind limb.

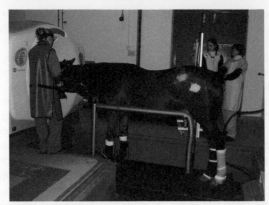

Fig. 2. A horse is positioned on a hovercraft table for standing, sedated skull CT examination at Royal Veterinary College, University of London, United Kingdom.

A CT scan series is a set of cross-sectional images, contiguous or overlapping, that represents a volume of tissue. Each volume element (voxel) is assigned a numerical value that is based on the tissue density relative to water. The numerical value is also termed a Hounsfield (HU) or CT unit, and the value of pure water is arbitrarily set to HU = 0.

The volumetric data that are acquired can be manipulated in many different ways, including preprocessing, postprocessing, multiplanar reconstruction, and 3D rendering.

Preprocessing occurs at the level of the CT scanner and is generally incorporated into the acquisition step. Preprocessing can account for systematic inconsistencies in the imaging equipment as well as noise within the images. The images can be then further processed by mathematically manipulating the data to emphasize or deemphasize certain aspects of the image characteristics. The mathematical model is termed an algorithm. For example, if an image made from raw or unfiltered data has a smooth or blurry appearance, the data can then be manipulated to sharpen the image or emphasize edges, a common technique in the evaluation of bone (**Fig. 3**).[2,3]

Postprocessing is image manipulation that occurs, in general, by the end-user. This broad term encompasses many aspects of image manipulation that vary from altering window width and level (analogous to brightness and contrast), to multiplanar reformatting, to 3D volume or surface rendering of the data set to evaluate tissues of similar density or surfaces respectively. Most Digital Imaging and Communication in Medicine (DICOM; NEMA, Rosslyn, VA, USA) viewer software programs (eg, eFilm, OsiriX) have the ability to perform basic manipulations of the information, but for some more complicated tasks, greater computing power is required. Thus, many rendering tasks are often performed on a dedicated workstation with more powerful, often proprietary software. All basic viewers of these programs will allow for manipulation of window width and level. A wide window width is appropriate for the evaluation of tissues with a broad variation in inherent tissue density such as bone ($\sim$400–1500 HU), whereas a narrow, or high contrast, window is more useful for tissues with little variation in tissue density such as tendons and ligaments ($\sim$40–120 HU). The term "level" refers to the center value of the window width. Altering level changes the brightness of the displayed image, and it should be manipulated routinely in image interpretation. Alteration of the window width and level by the end-user has no impact on the actual data set stored by the CT scanner.

Multiplanar reformatting allows the diagnostician to evaluate the anatomy in planes other than the axis of acquisition. This is a critically important tool because CT scans

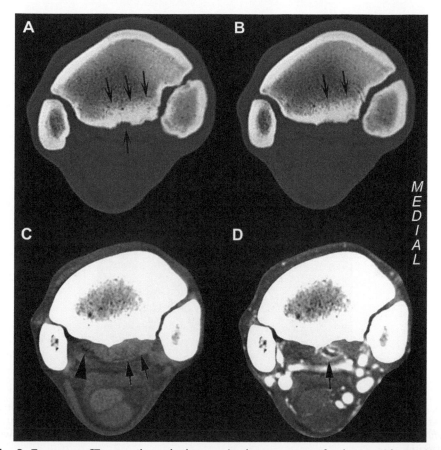

Fig. 3. Transverse CT scans through the proximal metacarpus of a horse with proximal suspensory desmopathy/enthesopathy. (*A, B*) The images are displayed with a bone window (width = 1600, level = 500) and are processed using an edge-enhancing algorithm. There is sclerosis on the endosteal surface (*black open arrows*) of the palmar cortex of the proximal third metacarpal bone, deep to the proximal suspensory ligament attachment. (*C, D*) The images are displayed using a soft tissue window (width = 400 HU, level = 150 HU) and processed with a smoothing algorithm. (*C*) Precontrast, transverse CT scan that shows normal, low-density adipose and muscular tissue of the lateral lobe of the proximal suspensory ligament (*black arrowhead*) and mild swelling, loss of the normal low-density adipose signal (*black arrows*). (*D*) Contrast, transverse CT scan at the same level shows moderate peripheral enhancement in the medial lobe of the proximal suspensory ligament (*black arrow*).

are always made perpendicular to the direction in which the anatomy passes through the gantry, regardless of positioning or conformation. Reformatting can be performed over a broad range from subtle, to correct for such things as patient conformation, to a complete rearrangement in image orientation from transverse to the sagittal, dorsal, or any oblique plane (**Fig. 4**). Reformatting is an integral part of image evaluation on a clinical level (**Fig. 5**). In addition to reslicing the data in alternative imaging planes, this technology can also be used to stack or add thin slices together to create an image of a "slab" of tissue. In doing so, the effect of image noise, meaning unwanted information within the image, can be reduced by increasing the desirable signal-to-noise ratio.

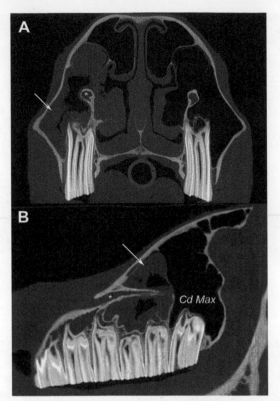

Fig. 4. Transverse (*A*) and parasagittal (*B*) images of a horse with rostral maxillary sinusitis. There is sinus mucosal thickening with soft tissue dense material accumulating in the rostral (*white arrows*) but not the caudal maxillary (Cd Max) sinus. The infraorbital canal is shown (*asterisk*).

Surface and volume rendering provide a 3D image of this area. In CT scanning, each voxel in the entire volume of tissue is assigned an HU or numerical value representing its relative density. This information is then used to produce 3D images. In surface rendering, the computer identifies edges of structures and their respective, assigned HU. Then using this as a threshold value, it eliminates the remaining tissues of different densities in the image, thus representing the surface only. This enables virtual endoscopy. Volume rendering is based on similar principles; the computer assigns a different color or shade (in the displayed image) to an HU range, thereby displaying a 3D volume with differentiation between the tissues. Furthermore, because the user can select the threshold values for color application and opacity, the user can then "remove" overlying tissues on the 3D model (**Fig. 6**). Clinically, this technique is very useful for understanding the surface configuration of fractures as a preoperative measure (**Fig. 7**) or understanding the relationship of the distal phalanx within the hoof capsule.

Contrast Media

Contrast agents are available for most diagnostic imaging modalities and are used to better identify or more thoroughly characterize either normal or pathologic structures. CT, as an x-ray–based technology, is amenable to the use of routine radiographic agents such as barium- or iodine-based substances.[1] Most often, iodinated, positive

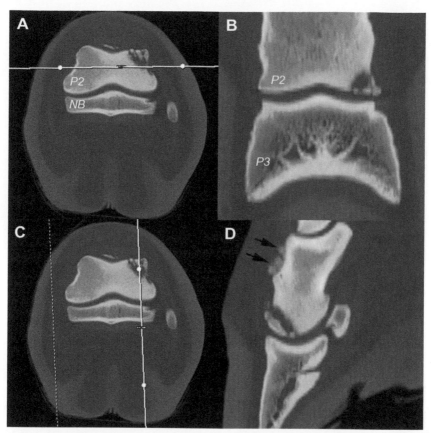

Fig. 5. Transverse (*A*, *C*) CT scans of a comminuted, articular fracture of the distal aspect of the middle phalanx. (*B*) Dorsal plane reformatted image through the fracture and the distal interphalangeal joint. (*A*) The white line denotes the reformatting plane and location. (*D*) A parasagittal reformatted scan through the fracture. There is irregular periosteal proliferation on the middle phalanx (*black arrows*). (*C*) The white line denotes the reformatting plane and location. NB, navicular (distal sesamoid) bone; P3, distal phalanx; P2, middle phalanx.

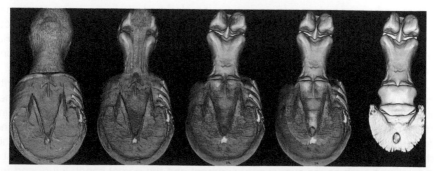

Fig. 6. Three-dimensional volume-rendered images of a horse with infection of the distal phalanx and a draining tract through the sole. Software is used to assign colors to tissues of similar density. From left to right, the superficial structures have been progressively removed, allowing the viewer to see that the defect in the distal phalanx is in a slightly different location than the defect in the hoof surface.

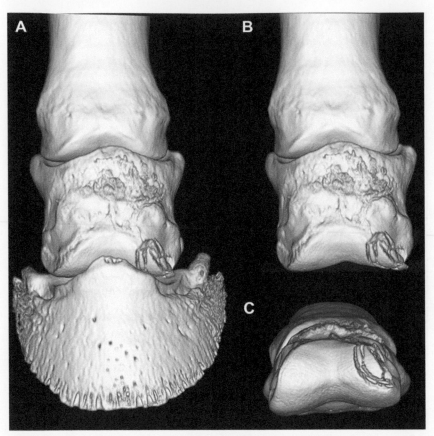

Fig. 7. Three-dimensional surface-rendered images of the phalanges of a horse with a middle phalanx, comminuted articular fracture, shown in **Fig. 5**. (*A*) Dorsal view of the phalanges showing the fracture and the irregular periosteal proliferation and the dorsal aspect of the middle phalanx. (*B*) Dorsal view of the middle phalanx and software has been used to select and remove the distal phalanx from the image. (*C*) Distal view of the articular surface of the middle phalanx.

contrast media are administered via an intravascular[4] and intra-articular[5–7] injection in the horse. Ionic and nonionic products are available. Only nonionic iodinated products are appropriate for use in synovial and subarachnoid spaces. In horses, intra-arterial infusion of ionic contrast media frequently results in minor but measurable alterations in blood pressure and heart rate.[8]

Contrast agents, when administered via an intravascular route, identify tissues with abnormally increased or decreased blood flow or regions with altered vascular permeability, as expected with injured or inflamed soft tissues. Regional intra-arterial administration of contrast media to the equine foot aids in soft tissue lesion identification and characterization.[4,9] Although more commonly used for foot-related lameness, this technique can be modified for the evaluation of more proximal regions in the hindlimbs and forelimbs such as the suspensory ligament and the carpal canal. Injury and the reparative processes associated with tendon and ligament pathologic conditions provide accumulation of contrast media in tissues by extravasation from abnormally permeable blood vessels. As a lesion repairs or responds to injury, new blood vessels develop and contrast media is seen within small-caliber blood vessels.[10]

CT arthrography (bursography) is performed by injecting nonionic iodine-based contrast media into synovial spaces to surround and improve margin visibility of structures in or around joints, sheaths, and bursae. This increases the diagnostic utility of the technique by providing a means of evaluating intra-articular ligaments (stifle, carpus) and identifying adhesions (navicular bursa) or articular or fibrocartilage cartilage lesions. CT arthrography of the stifle has greatly increased the diagnostic capabilities for this large, complicated joint.[5,6,11]

Advances in Clinical Use of CT

The clinical uses of CT are numerous and varied. The body of knowledge surrounding the use of CT and its applications continues to expand as more institutions and private practices put the technology to the test. Critical evaluation of clinical and research applications for the technology are being reported on with increasing frequency.

LAMENESS DIAGNOSIS
Foot

CT and intra-arterial CE-CT have been used as an alternative method to MR imaging for evaluating complex foot lameness in horses (**Fig. 8**).[4,10,12] Contrast delivery allows for the identification and characterization of tendon lesions, particularly when the lesions have evidence of healing by neovascularization.[10] CT has been described as superior to radiography for the identification of navicular degenerative changes, synovial invaginations, and distal border fragmentation.[13] CT has also been reported to be superior to MR imaging for the identification of osseous abnormalities in horses with foot lameness.[14,15]

Recent studies comparing CT and CE-CT to low field standing MR imaging in a cohort of horses with foot lameness showed some advantages of CT over MR imaging and some disadvantages.[16,17] CT had better image clarity at the margins of the imaging field and better bone imaging and better demonstrated sites of soft tissue and/or tendon mineralization. CT performed poorer than low field standing MR imaging for the evaluation of the deep digital flexor tendon over the face of the navicular bone and distal to the navicular bone. Also, by nature of the technique, CT does not identify STIR or T2 hyperintensity within bone, also termed "bone edema,"[16,17] a frequently implicated diagnostic imaging finding. In the study comparing lesion identification, most horses had a deep digital flexor tendon lesion and comparison of the imaging modalities in other soft tissue lesions was not performed.

Less information is available regarding the use of CT for the identification and characterization of other lesions in the foot. Presented but yet unpublished data from the University of California, Davis VMTH have shown a similar incidence of distal interphalangeal joint collateral ligament, collateral sesamoidean ligament, and navicular bone disease to other reports using high and/or low field MR imaging.[18–21] Furthermore, experience at this institution has demonstrated the clinical utility of the distal interphalangeal or metacarpophalangeal arthrography for the identification of full- or partial-thickness cartilage loss as a component of joint dysfunction (**Fig. 9**).

The role of CT in clinical laminitis management and laminitis research has not yet been defined. Dynamic CE-CT has been used to quantify blood flow to the foot in normal horses,[9] and this technique could be useful for the investigation of horses with laminitis or to evaluate the effect of medications or shoeing on digital blood flow. Clinically, CT aptly characterizes the osseous structures, hoof capsule, and, through vascular studies (arterial or venous), the laminar vasculature.

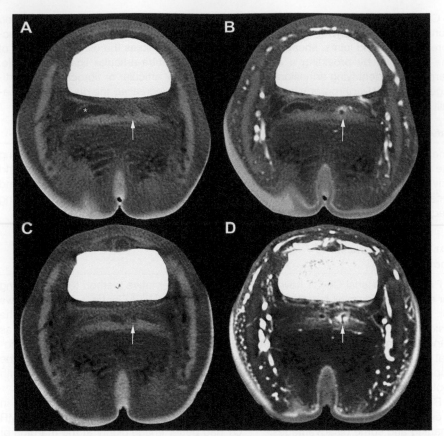

Fig. 8. Transverse precontrast (*A, C*) and postcontrast (*B, D*) images through the distal pastern of a horse with a deep digital flexor tendon (DDFT) tear (*white arrows*) at the level of the proximal reflection of the navicular bursa (*asterisk*). (*A, B*) Scans taken at the onset of lameness. The lesion in the DDFT is peripherally contrast enhancing. (*C, D*) Scans taken 11 months after the injury. There is increased enhancement, indicating increased blood flow with decreased size of the central, nonenhancing portion.

Tarsus/Stifle

CT and CT arthrography have been described and used in lameness diagnosis when the lameness is localized to the tarsus and the stifle.[5–7,11] In the tarsus, CT is useful for the diagnosis of occult joint disease, the characterization of traumatic lesions including fracture of the tarsal or metatarsal bones,[22] and the identification of other joint region osseous lesions such as subchondral osseous cyst–like lesions (**Fig. 10**).[23] In the stifle, CT arthrography has been used for the diagnosis of many soft tissue and periarticular osseous lesions resulting from performance related injuries, degeneration, or developmental orthopedic disease. The pathologic change identified includes injury of the cruciate ligaments, menisci, meniscal ligaments, cartilage, and subchondral bone[6] (Bergman and Puchalski, personal communication, 2012).

Other

The use of CT in equine lameness diagnosis extends beyond these specific and reported applications, and CT can be used as an adjunct test for any anatomic region

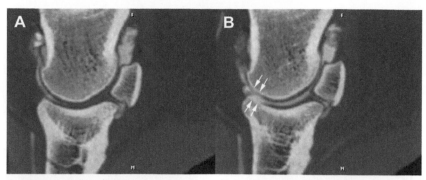

Fig. 9. Contrast arthrogram of the distal interphalangeal joint of a horse with full-thickness cartilage loss on the dorsal aspect of the joint (*white arrows*). (*A*) Parasagittal image of the lateral aspect of the joint. (*B*) Parasagittal image of the medial aspect of the joint. Synovial fluid is mixed with positive contrast medially and shows as white on the image. Synovial fluid is in contact with the subchondral bone of the distal dorsal aspect of the middle phalanx and the proximal dorsal aspect of the distal phalanx, documenting cartilage loss.

that can be scanned. CT is reported for the characterization of proximal suspensory enthesis new bone formation.[24] The addition of regional, intra-arterial contrast media can aid in the identification and also the characterization of suspensory desmopathy in the fore and hindlimbs (**Fig. 11**). Furthermore, CT has been useful for the identification of lesions involving the palmar carpal and intercarpal ligaments (**Fig. 12**). Carpal arthrography shows promise as a clinically applicable technique to identify palmar, intercarpal and cartilage injury in the carpus (Gray, Puchalski unpublished data).

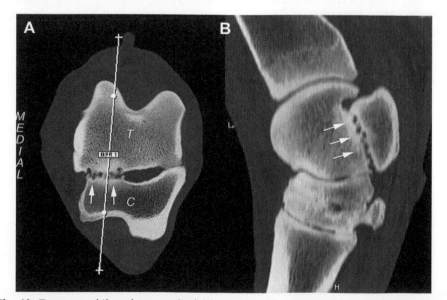

Fig. 10. Transverse (*A*) and parasagittal (*B*) CT scans of a tarsus with irregular bone lysis, proliferation, and partial ankylosis of the medial aspect of the talocalcaneal joint (*white arrows*). T, talus; C, calcaneus.

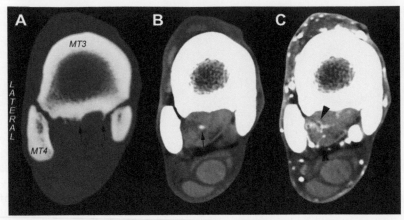

Fig. 11. Transverse CT scans through the proximal metatarsus identifying proximal suspensory desmopathy/enthesopathy. (*A*) The bone window aids in the identification of irregular bone proliferation (*black arrows*) associated with the medial and lateral proximal attachment of the suspensory ligament. (*B*) The soft tissue window demonstrates enlargement and partial mineralization (*black arrow*) of the proximal suspensory ligament. (*C*) The postcontrast, soft tissue window demonstrates enhancement of the suspensory ligament with an internal focus of nonenhancing hypodense ligament (*black arrowhead*). MT4, fourth metatarsal bone, MT3, third metatarsal bone.

Fetlock

Fetlock pathologic conditions are an important problem in equine lameness diagnosis. Earlier detection or more sensitive tests for fetlock pathologic conditions will serve veterinary medicine well, particularly in the thoroughbred racehorse. Several studies exist discussing the merits of CT for the diagnosis of early joint disease, developmental orthopedic disease, and subchondral bone injury.[25–30] The technique has

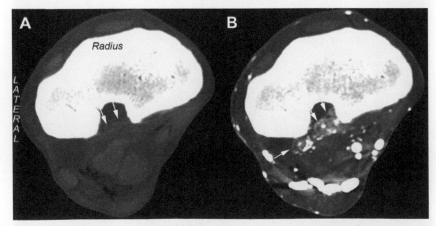

Fig. 12. Transverse scans at the level of the distal radius. These images document enlargement, irregular margination, and diffuse contrast enhancement of the common palmar carpal ligament and the palmar ligament between the radius and radial carpal bone (*white arrows*).

been used clinically but also as an invaluable research tool to better understand the underlying pathologic change in osteoarthritis,[25,27,28] condylar fracture,[31,32] and third metacarpal palmar condyle disease.[25] In osteoarthritis, CT consistently identified lesions of the noncartilaginous structures including osteophytes, subchondral sclerosis, lysis, osseous cyst–like lesions, and joint effusion better than orthogonal radiographs.[27] In this study, CT and MR imaging were used to identify and describe a relatively novel finding in equine osteoarthritis termed central, subchondral osteophytes, whereby new bone formation extends from the subchondral bone into the overlying cartilage. CT and MR imaging identified these osteophytes more often than radiography, and the osteophytes were associated with overlying cartilage damage identified on gross inspection.[28] In horses with severe condylar fractures, CT was shown to better identify additional sites of pathologic change than radiographs including abnormalities of the surrounding subchondral bone, sesamoid bones, and proximal phalanx.[31] In the evaluation of articular injury to the distal third metacarpal bone, CT and MR imaging identified sites of subchondral bone pathologic change but CT did not identify sites of cartilage degeneration.[25] Neither CT nor MR imaging identified sites of cartilage cracking.[25] However, there was a high correlation between sites of subchondral bone damage, as seen on imaging studies, and overlying articular cartilage damage, as seen on gross inspection.[25]

PREOPERATIVE PLANNING

As an extension of its role in lameness diagnosis, CT is used for preoperative planning for foot surgery[33] and fracture repair.[31,34,35] CT has often been described as a benefit in preoperative or intraoperative management of fractures (**Fig. 13**). The cross-sectional nature of the modality enables a very detailed evaluation of the fracture configuration that is superior to plain radiography. Modern software also allows for

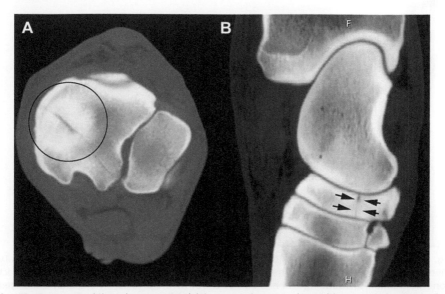

Fig. 13. Transverse (*A*) and parasagittal (*B*) scans of a central tarsal bone slab fracture. The fracture line propagates through a region of sclerosis not identified on radiographs (*black circle*).

3D reconstruction of the information to represent the imaging data in a manner more similar to that seen by surgeons during surgery.

SKULL AND DENTAL DISEASE

CT is very useful for the diagnosis and characterization of diseases of the equine skull, including the nasal passages, paranasal sinuses, and dentition. CT easily documents pathologic change of dental, osseous, and soft tissues in the skull, and there is increasing knowledge in this field of study.[36–50] CT is also useful for the characterization of some intracranial diseases[38,43] but is considered less desirable than MR imaging for brain imaging. Similar to other locations, CT has been a great asset as a research tool for furthering the global understanding of disease processes of the skull.

DENTAL DISEASE

There are clinical and research applications of CT for equine dental disease. The use of this modality has led to a greater understanding of abnormalities of the cheek teeth, particularly when accompanied by infectious and inflammatory complications like osteomyelitis and sinusitis. Descriptive reports have provided imaging findings of abnormalities of dental components, surrounding alveoli, and supporting bone structures and the sinuses.[39,49] These reports identify CT imaging findings such as hypoattenuation of cementum, dentin, and enamel in concert with widening of the pulp, gas accumulation and tooth root bulging, fragmentation, and periapical abscessation (**Fig. 14**). The aforementioned descriptive study documented common findings with dental disease–associated sinusitis, including maxillary bone reaction, sinus epithelial thickening, and involvement of the infraorbital canal and frontomaxillary aperture.[49] Further work was initiated to answer more questions regarding internal endodontal anatomy and disease pathogenesis. A more recent study capitalized on the ability

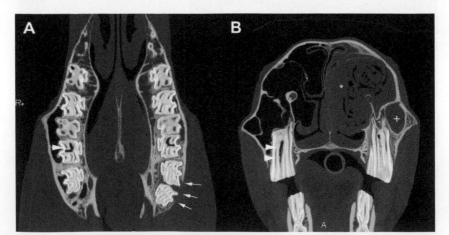

Fig. 14. Dorsal (A) and transverse (B) scans of a horse with a supranumerary left maxillary cheek tooth (*white arrows*). (A) The second premolars are not included. There is compact bone destruction surrounding this anomalous tooth (*white arrows*). There is an associated abscess in the left maxillary sinus (*asterisk*) containing inspissated inflammatory material and feed. The rostral maxillary sinus is full of fluid (+). This horse has infundibular gas and probable necrosis of the second maxillary molars (110, 210) (*arrowheads*).

of CT to provide 3D models with segmentation by tissue density to further understand the internal architecture of dental pulp, including pulpar communications and infundibulae.[44] This work went on to describe several important, normal, age-related changes in dental and pulp morphology. This same group further evaluated and described cheek teeth with occlusal and CT abnormalities, finding a very high incidence of infundibular abnormalities, citing this as evidence to support the clinical significance of infundibular decay.[45] A different group used CT in horses with and without dental abnormalities. This group found that CT was necessary to fully evaluate the infundibula and that abnormal infundibula could not be statistically associated with apical abnormalities. They further suggested that no conclusions can be made if infundibular abnormalities are identified on CT.[46] Practically, CT is an excellent tool that can evaluate the internal architecture of teeth and their surrounding environment without the problem of superimposition present on routine projectional radiographs.

TEMPOROHYOID OSTEOARTHROPATHY

CT is an invaluable adjunct diagnostic modality to radiography and sinoscopy for the characterization of a variety of nondental pathologic conditions of the skull including temporohyoid osteoarthropathy (THO) and skull fractures.[39,41–43,50,51] THO is particularly amenable to evaluation with CT scanning because of the high variability in tissue density (air of guttural pouch to petrous temporal bone). CT has led to a greater understanding of the extent and severity of involvement of the temporal bone, including the osseous bullae, and the hyoid apparatus, including the stylohyoid and ceratohyoid bones.[50] CT provides additional information to radiography and endoscopy by identifying temporal and ceratohyoid bone changes not previously described. Peripheral quantitative CT, a technique similar to clinical CT, has been used as research tool to identify age associated degeneration of the temporohyoid joint and to propose degenerative disease as an cause of THO.[42] In the same anatomic region, the identification of fractures, often associated with cranial nerve VII and VIII deficits, can be difficult or impossible with routine radiography.[41,51] The identification of fractures in this region is an excellent indication for CT; however, care must be taken to accurately interpret the numerous foramina and fissura of the region. An anatomic guide to CT scans of the equine temporal bone has now been published to aid in this endeavor.[41] Similarly, CT is very useful to fully characterize traumatic lesions of the mandible.[39]

SINONASAL DISEASE

Mass lesions of the equine nasal passages and paranasal sinuses, including ethmoid hematoma and neoplasia, can be challenging to treat and diagnose. Sinoscopy, endoscopy, and radiography are useful but may underestimate or incompletely characterize these lesions. A retrospective study evaluating the impact of CT findings on treatment or prognosis showed that ethmoid hematoma occurred bilaterally, involved the paranasal sinuses including the sphenopalatine sinuses in many horses, and was associated with other sinonasal disease in some cases.[36] This study also described that 63% of ethmoid hematomas had a hyperattenuating swirling pattern that likely relates to partial mineralization identified on histopathologic examination (**Fig. 15**).[36] In contrast, a study evaluating a group of sinonasal tumors of variable tissue origin showed that most tumors were homogeneous and of soft tissue density on CT scans.[40] This report further showed that the vast majority of these tumors were associated with moderate or marked osseous destruction of the nasal or ethmoturbinates or compact bone of the skull.[40] This study also had a surprising distribution of tumors

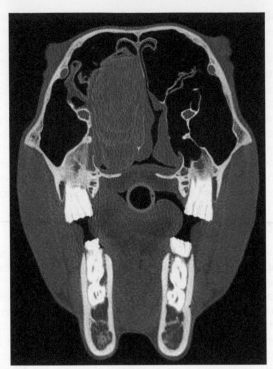

Fig. 15. Transverse CT scan of an ethmoid hematoma with an internal swirling hyperattenuating pattern. The lesion is immediately adjacent to the infraorbital canal.

with several being neuroendocrine/neuroblastomas.[40] Publications about paranasal sinus cysts are still lacking.

INTRACRANIAL DISEASE

CT provides useful information for many but not all intracranial lesions. A recent report has evaluated the diagnostic utility of the technique for a variety of intracranial disorders ranging from malignant neoplasia to skull trauma.[43] Evaluated the accuracy of this tool using histopathologic and gross pathologic examinations as gold standard tests and found high specificity but moderate (57%) sensitivity compared with histopathologic examination. CT did have a high sensitivity compared with gross pathologic examination alone. CT readily identified hemorrhage, fractures, and parenchymal lesions causing mass effect (brain tumors). CT and even C-E CT failed to identify meningitis and small brain parenchymal lesions.[43] CT also proved useful for the characterization of pituitary pars intermedia dysfunction whereby CT provided accurate measurements of the pituitary dimensions and therefore volume that correlated well with pituitary gland weight measured postmortem.[38]

SUMMARY

CT is a valid and useful technique for the characterization and investigation of many, variable disease processes in equine practice. This technique is limited only by patient size, hardware considerations, and the end-users' imaginations. Great advances have been made in hardware including CT scanner gantries and equine tables, software, and the greater body of knowledge. Like all things, as global understanding of the technique and its capabilities increases, so does the need for further investigation.

REFERENCES

1. Bushberg J, Seibert J, Leidholdt E, et al. The essential physics of medical imaging. 2nd edition. Philadelphia: Lippincott, Williams and Wilkins; 2002.
2. Cody DD. Image processing in CT. Radiographics 2002;22:1255–68.
3. Lo WY, Puchalski SM. Digital image processing. Vet Radiol Ultrasound 2008;49: S42–7.
4. Puchalski SM, Galuppo LD, Hornof WJ, et al. Intraarterial contrast-enhanced computed tomography of the equine distal extremity. Vet Radiol Ultrasound 2007;48:21–9.
5. Vekens EV, Bergman EH, Vanderperren K, et al. Computed tomographic anatomy of the equine stifle joint. Am J Vet Res 2011;72:512–21.
6. Bergman HJ, Puchalski SM, van der Veen H, et al. Computed tomography and CT arthrography of the equine stifle: technique and preliminary results in 16 clinical cases. Lexington: American Association of Equine Practitioners; 2007. 46–55.
7. Raes EV, Bergman EH, van der Veen H, et al. Comparison of cross-sectional anatomy and computed tomography of the tarsus in horses. Am J Vet Res 2011;72:1209–21.
8. Pollard RE, Puchalski SM. Reaction to intraarterial ionic iodinated contrast medium administration in anesthetized horses. Vet Radiol Ultrasound 2011;52: 441–3.
9. Kruger EF, Puchalski SM, Pollard RE, et al. Measurement of equine laminar blood flow and vascular permeability by use of dynamic contrast-enhanced computed tomography. Am J Vet Res 2008;69:371–7.
10. Puchalski SM, Galuppo LD, Drew CP, et al. Use of contrast-enhanced computed tomography to assess angiogenesis in deep digital flexor tendonopathy in a horse. Vet Radiol Ultrasound 2009;50:292–7.
11. Crijns CP, Gielen IM, van Bree HJ, et al. The use of CT and CT arthrography in diagnosing equine stifle injury in a Rheinlander gelding. Equine Vet J 2010;42: 367–71.
12. Puchalski SM, Snyder JR, Hornof WJ, et al. Contrast enhanced computed tomography of the equine distal extremity. Lexington: AAEP Proceedings. 2005.
13. Claerhoudt S, Bergman HJ, Van Der Veen H, et al. Differences in the morphology of distal border synovial invaginations of the distal sesamoid bone in the horse as evaluated by computed tomography compared with radiography. Equine Vet J 2012. http://dx.doi.org/10.1111/j.2042-3306.2012.00547.x.
14. Widmer WR, Buckwalter KA, Fessler JF, et al. Use of radiography, computed tomography and magnetic resonance imaging for evaluation of navicular syndrome in the horse. Vet Radiol Ultrasound 2000;41:108–16.
15. Whitton RC, Buckley C, Donovan T, et al. The diagnosis of lameness associated with distal limb pathology in a horse: a comparison of radiography, computed tomography and magnetic resonance imaging. Vet J 1998;155:223–9.
16. Vallance SA, Bell RJ, Spriet M, et al. Comparisons of computed tomography, contrast enhanced computed tomography and standing low-field magnetic resonance imaging in horses with lameness localised to the foot. Part 1: anatomic visualisation scores. Equine Vet J 2012;44:51–6.
17. Vallance SA, Bell RJ, Spriet M, et al. Comparisons of computed tomography, contrast-enhanced computed tomography and standing low-field magnetic

resonance imaging in horses with lameness localised to the foot. Part 2: lesion identification. Equine Vet J 2012;44:149–56.

18. Puchalski SM, Schultz RM, Bell RJ, et al. Intra-arterial contrast enhanced computed tomography in equine foot lameness: 151 horses. American College of Veterinary Radiology Annual Conference. Memphis, September, 2009.

19. Dyson S, Murray R. Magnetic resonance imaging evaluation of 264 horses with foot pain: the podotrochlear apparatus, deep digital flexor tendon and collateral ligaments of the distal interphalangeal joint. Equine Vet J 2007;39:340–3.

20. Mair TS, Kinns J. Deep digital flexor tendonitis in the equine foot diagnosed by low-field magnetic resonance imaging in the standing patient: 18 cases. Vet Radiol Ultrasound 2005;46:458–66.

21. Sampson SN, Schneider RK, Gavin PR, et al. Magnetic resonance imaging findings in horses with recent onset navicular syndrome but without radiographic abnormalities. Vet Radiol Ultrasound 2009;50:339–46.

22. Poulin-Braim AE, Bell RJ, Textor J, et al. Computed tomography of proximal metatarsal and concurrent third tarsal bone fractures in a thoroughbred racehorse. Equine Vet Educ 2010;22:290–5.

23. Garcia-Lopez JM, Kirker-Head CA. Occult subchondral osseous cyst-like lesions of the equine tarsocrural joint. Vet Surg 2004;33:557–64.

24. Launois MT, Vandeweerd JM, Perrin RA, et al. Use of computed tomography to diagnose new bone formation associated with desmitis of the proximal aspect of the suspensory ligament in third metacarpal or third metatarsal bones of three horses. J Am Vet Med Assoc 2009;234:514–8.

25. O'Brien T, Baker TA, Brounts SH, et al. Detection of articular pathology of the distal aspect of the third metacarpal bone in thoroughbred racehorses: comparison of radiography, computed tomography and magnetic resonance imaging. Vet Surg 2011;40:942–51.

26. Olive J, d'Anjou MA, Alexander K, et al. Correlation of signal attenuation-based quantitative magnetic resonance imaging with quantitative computed tomographic measurements of subchondral bone mineral density in metacarpophalangeal joints of horses. Am J Vet Res 2010;71:412–20.

27. Olive J, D'Anjou MA, Alexander K, et al. Comparison of magnetic resonance imaging, computed tomography, and radiography for assessment of noncartilaginous changes in equine metacarpophalangeal osteoarthritis. Vet Radiol Ultrasound 2010;51:267–79.

28. Olive J, D'Anjou MA, Girard C, et al. Imaging and histological features of central subchondral osteophytes in racehorses with metacarpophalangeal joint osteoarthritis. Equine Vet J 2009;41:859–64.

29. Vanderperren K, Ghaye B, Snaps FR, et al. Evaluation of computed tomographic anatomy of the equine metacarpophalangeal joint. Am J Vet Res 2008;69:631–8.

30. Schoenborn WC, Rick MC, Hornof WJ. Computed tomographic appearance of osteochondritis dissecans-like lesions of the proximal articular surface of the proximal phalanx in a horse. Vet Radiol Ultrasound 2002;43:541–4.

31. Morgan JW, Santschi EM, Zekas LJ, et al. Comparison of radiography and computed tomography to evaluate metacarpo/metatarsophalangeal joint pathology of paired limbs of thoroughbred racehorses with severe condylar fracture. Vet Surg 2006;35:611–7.

32. Whitton RC, Trope GD, Ghasem-Zadeh A, et al. Third metacarpal condylar fatigue fractures in equine athletes occur within previously modelled subchondral bone. Bone 2010;47:826–31.

33. Getman LM, Davidson EJ, Ross MW, et al. Computed tomography or magnetic resonance imaging-assisted partial hoof wall resection for keratoma removal. Vet Surg 2011;40:708–14.

34. Waselau M, Bertone AL, Green EM. Computed tomographic documentation of a comminuted fourth carpal bone fracture associated with carpal instability treated by partial carpal arthrodesis in an Arabian filly. Vet Surg 2006;35:618–25.

35. Rose PL, Seeherman H, O'Callaghan M. Computed tomographic evaluation of comminuted middle phalangeal fractures in the horse. Vet Radiol Ultrasound 1997;38:424–9.

36. Textor J, Puchalski SM, Affolter VK, et al. Computed tomographic findings in ethmoid hematoma: impact on treatment and outcome (16 cases, 1993–2005). JAVMA 2012;240(11):1338–44.

37. Scrivani PV. Advanced imaging of the nervous system in the horse. Vet Clin North Am Equine Pract 2011;27:439–53.

38. Pease AP, Schott HC 2nd, Howey EB, et al. Computed tomographic findings in the pituitary gland and brain of horses with pituitary pars intermedia dysfunction. J Vet Intern Med 2011;25:1144–51.

39. Huggons NA, Bell RJ, Puchalski SM. Radiography and computed tomography in the diagnosis of nonneoplastic equine mandibular disease. Vet Radiol Ultrasound 2011;52:53–60.

40. Cissell DD, Wisner ER, Textor J, et al. Computed tomographic appearance of equine sinonasal neoplasia. Vet Radiol Ultrasound 2012;53(3):245–51.

41. Pownder S, Scrivani PV, Bezuidenhout A, et al. Computed tomography of temporal bone fractures and temporal region anatomy in horses. J Vet Intern Med 2010;24:398–406.

42. Naylor RJ, Perkins JD, Allen S, et al. Histopathology and computed tomography of age-associated degeneration of the equine temporohyoid joint. Equine Vet J 2010;42:425–30.

43. Lacombe VA, Sogaro-Robinson C, Reed SM. Diagnostic utility of computed tomography imaging in equine intracranial conditions. Equine Vet J 2010;42:393–9.

44. Windley Z, Weller R, Tremaine WH, et al. Two- and three-dimensional computed tomographic anatomy of the enamel, infundibulae and pulp of 126 equine cheek teeth. Part 1: findings in teeth without macroscopic occlusal or computed tomographic lesions. Equine Vet J 2009;41:433–40.

45. Windley Z, Weller R, Tremaine WH, et al. Two- and three-dimensional computed tomographic anatomy of the enamel, infundibulae and pulp of 126 equine cheek teeth. Part 2: findings in teeth with macroscopic occlusal or computed tomographic lesions. Equine Vet J 2009;41:441–7.

46. Veraa S, Voorhout G, Klein WR. Computed tomography of the upper cheek teeth in horses with infundibular changes and apical infection. Equine Vet J 2009;41:872–6.

47. Rodriguez MJ, Latorre R, Lopez-Albors O, et al. Computed tomographic anatomy of the temporomandibular joint in the young horse. Equine Vet J 2008;40:566–71.

48. Probst A, Henninger W, Willmann M. Communications of normal nasal and paranasal cavities in computed tomography of horses. Vet Radiol Ultrasound 2005;46:44–8.

49. Henninger W, Frame EM, Willmann M, et al. CT features of alveolitis and sinusitis in horses. Vet Radiol Ultrasound 2003;44:269–76.

50. Hilton H, Puchalski SM, Aleman M. The computed tomographic appearance of equine temporohyoid osteoarthropathy. Vet Radiol Ultrasound 2009;50:151–6.

51. Walker AM, Sellon DC, Cornelisse CJ, et al. Temporohyoid osteoarthropathy in 33 horses (1993–2000). J Vet Intern Med 2002;16:697–703.

Computed Tomographic Arthrography of the Equine Stifle Joint

Alejandro Valdés-Martínez, MVZ

KEYWORDS

- Stifle • Computed tomography • Arthrography • CTR • Multiplanar reconstruction

KEY POINTS

- Stifle computed tomographic arthrography (CTR) is a useful technique for evaluation of the internal soft tissue structures of the joint.
- The quality of a CTR examination is highly technique dependent; therefore, areas within the joint that are not outlined by contrast medium are difficult to evaluate and often result in a nondiagnostic study.
- Soft tissue architectural changes and lesions communicating with the joint space due to damage to the periphery of the soft tissues or articular cartilage/subchondral bone are general categories of pathologic conditions that can be diagnosed with CTR.
- Stifle CTR complements other diagnostic imaging modalities and arthroscopy to achieve a thorough evaluation of the joint.

INTRODUCTION

Arthrography is a diagnostic imaging technique that was used for many decades to enhance visualization of intraarticular structures not apparent on plain radiography. As ultrasonography and magnetic resonance imaging (MRI) became more available in veterinary medicine, the use of arthrography declined. Ultrasonography and MRI have become the modalities of choice for imaging soft tissues. However, like any imaging modality, both have advantages and disadvantages.

Ultrasonography is used frequently to diagnose many musculoskeletal diseases in horses, including pathologic changes affecting the stifle. Advantages of this modality include the ability to perform the examination on a standing horse and consequently an understanding of positional abnormalities can be accomplished using dynamic examination with flexion and extension of the limb. Furthermore, if performed by a skilled sonographer, the results of a stifle ultrasound examination are usually

The author has nothing to disclose.
Department of Environmental and Radiological Health Sciences, College of Veterinary Medicine and Biomedical Sciences, Colorado State University, 300 West Drake Road, Fort Collins, CO 80523-1620, USA
E-mail address: avaldes@colostate.edu

rewarding. However, limitations of ultrasonography of the equine stifle joint exist and are well documented.[1]

MRI gives excellent contrast resolution of soft tissues and provides multiple plane visualization of all anatomic structures that comprise the stifle joint. Unfortunately, MRI of the equine stifle is limited due to magnet bore diameter and length. Most MR systems do not allow the limb to be placed far enough into the magnet to image the stifle properly. In addition, MRI has the greatest anesthesia time and cost when compared with other modalities.

Computed tomography (CT) has been used increasingly in some veterinary institutions for the evaluation of the equine appendicular skeleton, including the stifle joint. CT images are obtained in the transverse plane. The computer can then create images in any other plane required to evaluate the anatomic region further. The images are called multiplanar reconstructions (MPR). In the last few years, the development of helical scanners with multiple rows of detectors has resulted in much faster scan times. In addition, the capability of submillimetric image acquisition and isotropic (identical spatial resolution in all dimensions) or near isotropic reconstructions has greatly improved the spatial resolution on MPR images. Unfortunately, visualization of the soft tissues with CT is limited and commonly unrewarding without the use of intravascular or intraarticular contrast. Computed tomographic arthrography (CTR) is an imaging technique that uses intraarticular administration of contrast to improve visualization of the intrasynovial and perisynovial soft tissue structures. The contrast medium will diffuse within the joint compartments, making the soft tissue structures more conspicuous. The soft tissue structures appear as filling defects outlined by the contrast in the joint. CTR is used to identify abnormalities in the articular surfaces, intrasynovial soft tissue structures, synovial surface of the joint capsule, and periarticular structures that have a close relationship with the joint compartments. Abnormalities in the size, shape, or margins of the intrasynovial soft tissue structures are identified because of an abnormal contrast pattern. The contrast will outline structures and reveal abnormalities in size and shape. Contrast will enter tears or defects, demonstrating injury to soft tissue structures or articular surfaces.

The terminology used in CT and CTR when describing a particular anatomic structure or lesion will depend on the attenuation (density) of that structure in relation to the surrounding tissue. Hyperattenuating means that the structure being described is denser (brighter) than the surrounding tissue. Hypoattenuating means that the structure being described is less dense (darker) than the surrounding tissue, and isoattenuating means that the densities are the same. These terms can also be used by applying a direct comparison, eg, the cranial cruciate ligament is hypoattenuating to cortical bone.

CLINICAL INDICATIONS FOR STIFLE CTR

Once the source of lameness is localized to the stifle joint, noninvasive diagnostic techniques such as radiography and ultrasonography are commonly used for further evaluation of the joint. However both modalities have limitations, and occasionally the findings seen with the combination of these 2 modalities may not be sufficient to explain the results of the lameness examination. Whereas stifle arthroscopy is often performed as the next diagnostic step and has been considered the gold standard for evaluation of the internal joint structures, it has limitations for visualization of some regions within the joint.[1,2]

Stifle CT allows visualization of the joint, giving excellent information regarding bony changes. With the addition of CTR, the ability for evaluating the internal soft tissue structures is greatly increased. Stifle CTR is indicated in cases with lameness localized to the stifle that cannot be explained by other imaging modalities (radiography and/or ultrasound), and when a better understanding of the internal condition of the joint is needed for case management and prognosis.

PATIENT PREPARATION AND INJECTION TECHNIQUE

After induction of anesthesia, the patient is placed on the CT table in lateral recumbency position with the affected stifle on the dependent side; that leg is extended in line with the patient table (**Fig. 1**). General anesthesia should be maintained with either injectable or gas anesthetics. The area for arthrocentesis should be aseptically prepared before the injection. If needed, the hair can be clipped before aseptic preparation of the injection sites.

Different techniques for arthrocentesis of the stifle joint have been described and include a 3-injection technique with placement of an 18-gauge 1.5-in needle in each individual compartment, or a single approach technique using an 18-gauge 3.5-in needle for all 3 compartments.[3] If needed, ultrasound-guided injection of each individual compartment may be used for accurate contrast medium administration.[4]

At our institution, a modified technique consisting of the single approach with an additional individual injection of the medial femorotibial joint compartment has resulted in adequate contrast distribution in the stifle. This modified technique consists of inserting an 18-gauge 3.5-in spinal needle between the middle and medial patellar ligaments midway between the distal patella and the proximal aspect of the tibial tuberosity. The needle is directed caudolaterally and advanced to contact the axial aspect of the lateral femoral condyle in the lateral compartment of the femorotibial joint. Then the stylet is removed and the contrast medium is injected until back pressure is obtained. The stylet is then replaced and the needle is withdrawn to the subcutaneous tissue and redirected caudomedially to contact with the axial aspect of the medial femoral condyle within the medial compartment of the femorotibial joint. The injection procedure is then repeated as on the previous compartment. The stylet is

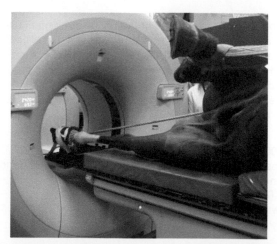

Fig. 1. Photograph showing the ideal positioning for CT of the equine stifle. The affected leg is positioned on the dependent side and placed as parallel as possible to the long axis of the patient table. The goal is to place the stifle joint as close to the isocenter of the CT gantry as possible. The opposite pelvic limb is flexed and pulled away from the gantry.

again replaced and the needle is withdrawn to the subcutaneous tissue and redirected proximally under the patella into the femoropatellar joint. Because of the lateral recumbency of the patient, the contrast medium may concentrate in the gravity-dependent lateral aspect of the femorotibial joint compartments. To assure the presence of contrast medium on the abaxial aspect of the medial femorotibial compartment, an additional injection of contrast medium with an 18-gauge 1.5-in needle placed between the medial patellar ligament and the medial collateral ligament is performed. The approach to the medial compartment can be easily assisted with ultrasound guidance.

The amount of contrast medium to be injected in the joint differs between patients and varies depending on the size of the synovial compartments, as well as the condition of the synovial lining and associated stretching ability of the capsule. Up to 360 mL (approximately 120 mL per synovial compartment) of contrast medium may be needed to achieve full distention in a 450-kg horse. After all the compartments are fully distended with contrast, the leg is flexed and extended several times to allow a uniform distribution of the contrast medium throughout the joint and for the contrast to diffuse into any soft tissue or bony defects that communicate with the joint space. The joint compartments should be decompressed as much as possible before anesthesia recovery.

CONTRAST MEDIUM

Iodinated contrast medium must be used for the arthrographic technique. Nonionic iodinated contrast medium is preferred because it is better tolerated by the joint than ionic iodinated contrast.[5] Many different products are available on the market, with the main difference being the concentration of iodine per milliliter. Regardless of the product used, the contrast medium should be diluted with sterile 0.9% physiologic saline solution (NaCl) to obtain a contrast medium with a minimum of 35 to 40 mg of iodine per milliliter. Concentrations of up to 150 mg iodine per milliliter have also provided successful results for equine stifle arthrography.[6]

CT PROTOCOL

The CT scanning protocol may vary depending on the equipment used and the size of the horse to be examined. Two scans obtained with different slice thicknesses and 2 algorithms (bone and standard or soft tissue) are ideal for evaluating bone and soft tissue structures. However, a viable option would be a single acquisition with thin slices; then the raw data of that acquisition is used to reformat it into thicker slices. In an average adult size horse (450–500 kg), the following image acquisition settings will provide adequate images for interpretation:

- kV: 120–140
- mAs: 400–500
- Slice thickness: 0.8–1.3 mm for adequate bone resolution and 1.5–2.0 mm to increase signal-to-noise ratio for soft tissue evaluation
- Pitch: 0.4–0.6
- Field-of-view: 35–45 cm
- Matrix: 512 × 512 to 1024×1024

PRINCIPLES OF IMAGE INTERPRETATION

Prearthography and postarthrography CT images should be assessed with a bone and a soft tissue window to allow proper evaluation of all structures comprising the stifle joint. MPR is an indispensable software tool available in the CT workstation and in most of the commercially available DICOM viewing software programs, which allows the images to be analyzed in all planes. Images can be reconstructed in transverse, sagittal, and frontal (coronal) planes with unlimited angle variation. It is critical to use MPR on all series acquired to manipulate the images in such a way that each structure is evaluated individually in multiple planes (**Fig. 2**). MPR is especially useful in the stifle to evaluate the cruciate ligaments, which run obliquely relative to the joint. A thorough comprehension of the internal anatomy of the equine stifle joint is necessary for an accurate interpretation.

Osseous Structures

Most pathologic changes in the bone detectable with CT are visible without the need of contrast medium. However, CTR is necessary to determine whether an osseous cystlike lesion in the subchondral bone communicates with the joint through a full-thickness cartilage defect. This type of cartilage/subchondral bone lesion is discussed in more detail later in this section.

Subchondral Bone Lesions

Subchondral bone lesions identified in the stifle using CT include subtle defects, cysts, or cystlike lesions. The medial femoral condyle is the most commonly affected region of subchondral bone in the stifle, and specifically, the cranial third of the condyle is the most frequently affected site (**Fig. 3**). Subchondral bone lesions may also appear on the lateral femoral condyle and medial and lateral tibial condyles. Another presentation of subchondral bone disease is the presence of patellar or trochlear ridge defects, most commonly seen as osteochondrosis or osteochondritis dissecans of the lateral trochlear ridge.

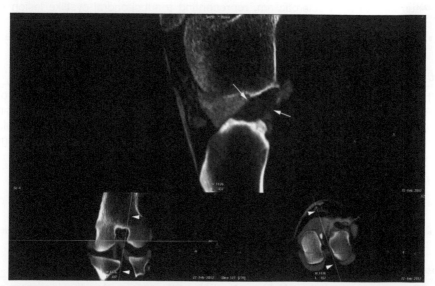

Fig. 2. Multiplanar reconstruction (MPR) images of a stifle CTR showing the cranial cruciate ligament on a sagittal plane (*arrows, top image*). Reference lines (*arrow heads*) on frontal (*bottom left*) and transverse (*bottom right*) plane images are used to align the sagittal plane along the longitudinal axis of the cranial cruciate ligament.

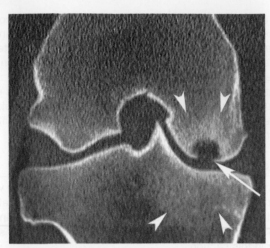

Fig. 3. Dorsal plane reconstruction showing a rounded lucent area (*arrow*) with surrounding sclerosis on the subchondral bone of the medial femoral condyle representing a cystlike lesion. Note the sclerosis surrounding the cystlike lesion and on the adjacent subchondral bone of the medial tibial condyle (*arrowheads*).

CT features of subchondral bone lesions

- Subtle loss of the normal smooth and uniformly continuous contour of the affected bone with a possible defect and surrounding sclerosis, representing a subchondral bone defect
- Well-defined, variably sized, rounded hypoattenuating areas near or in communication with the adjacent articular cartilage. These lesions may be also surrounded by a sclerotic rim, representing a subchondral cystlike lesion or osteochondrosis
- Well-defined, rounded osseous body associated with a trochlea ridge defect (osteochondritis dissecans)

Enthesopathy and Osteophytosis

Enthesopathy may be associated with or without a visible ligament or tendon injury on CTR and can be proliferative or resorptive (**Fig. 4**). Chronic resorption can result in osseous cyst-like lesions at soft tissue attachments, most commonly the cranial tibial meniscal ligaments. Osteophytes occur at the periarticular margins of the tibial and femoral condyles or patella and are secondary to a degenerative joint disease.

CT features of enthesopathy and osteophytosis

- Enthesopathy may be evident as irregular bone production, resorption, or a combination of both at the attachment of a soft tissue structure
- Osteophyte formation is normally seen as focal bony protrusions at the periarticular margins of the tibial and femoral condyles, and the patella

Trabecular Bone Lesions

On CT images, normal trabecular bone should have the same pattern that is present on radiographs, although it can be seen in greater detail. The hyperattenuating lines that make up the trabecular bone are usually oriented along the long axis of the bone, therefore are best visualized on sagittal or frontal reconstructions. Loss of the normal

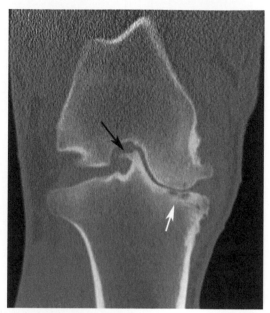

Fig. 4. Frontal plane reconstruction showing a decreased space between the medial femoral and the medial tibial condyles. There is evidence of adjacent subchondral bone erosion or "kissing lesions" between the femoral and tibial condyles (*white arrow*) with surrounding sclerosis. In addition, there is a prominent enthesophyte at the insertion of the cranial cruciate ligament on the medial intercondylar eminence of the tibia (*black arrow*). Also, a marked amount of periarticular osteophyte formation is evident along the medial aspect of the joint and enthesophytosis at the origin and insertion of the medial collateral ligament is present.

trabecular bone pattern can result from sclerosis, lysis, or a combination of both. Both sclerosis and lysis can occur simultaneously secondary to a chronic process, usually initiated or at least exacerbated by repetitive trauma, or may be secondary to an aggressive lesion, such as a septic process or neoplasia (**Fig. 5**).

CT features of trabecular bone sclerosis or lysis

- Sclerosis is evident as a hyperattenuating (white) region with increased bone density between the trabeculae, making it difficult to distinguish the normal trabecular pattern
- Lysis is evident as areas of bone loss and is usually irregular and with ill-defined margins

Fractures

Excellent assessment of complete fractures can be achieved with plain CT, MPR, and 3-dimensional reconstructions. Additional soft tissue injuries associated with the fracture can be assessed when performing CTR.

Incomplete, nondisplaced fractures and normal vascular channels can both appear as thin hypoattenuating lines on CT images. In addition, pathologic change in bone can be accompanied by a prominent vascular pattern with an increased number and the size of vascular channels. MPR is helpful for distinguishing between an incomplete, nondisplaced fracture and a vascular channel.

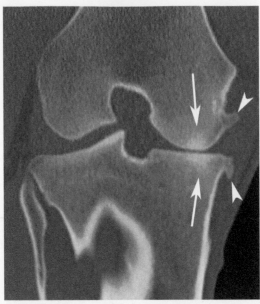

Fig. 5. Dorsal plane reconstruction showing a decreased space between the medial femoral and tibial condyles with additional hyperattenuating subchondral bone representing sclerosis (*arrows*) and likely a meniscal collapse and/or prolapse. Note the periarticular osteophyte formation on the medial aspect of the distal femur and proximal tibia (*arrowheads*).

- Incomplete, nondisplaced fractures appear as hypoattenuating (dark) fissures when evaluated on a plane perpendicular to the fracture line
- The fracture lines may be surrounded by abnormal bone depending on the cause (ie, fractures of sclerotic bone) and age (ie, old fractures with secondary sclerosis, widening of the fracture line, and/or periosteal new bone formation) of the fracture
- Vascular channels are cylindrical tracts and appear as circular hypoattenuating structures when evaluated on a plane perpendicular to the longitudinal axis of the vascular channel (**Fig. 6**A)
- Prominent vascular channels associated with abnormal bone are wide and usually extend from the periosteal surface and/or the physeal scar toward the periphery of the pathologic bone (see **Fig. 6**B, C)

Articular Cartilage

The articular surface is visible when contrast medium is in contact with the articular cartilage. The articular cartilage is evident as a smooth and uniform hypoattenuating line between the contrast medium and the subchondral bone (**Fig. 7**). To achieve this, the joint has to be fully distended and the contrast medium must cover the superficial margin of the articular cartilage completely.

Stifle CTR features of articular cartilage abnormalities

- Irregular interface between the contrast medium and the hypoattenuating (dark) line overlying the subchondral bone, thin hypoattenuating line, or contrast-filled surface defects in the hypoattenuating line, representing articular cartilage fraying, thinning, and/or partial thickness defects

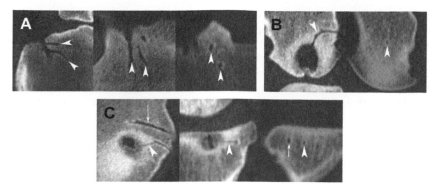

Fig. 6. (A) Sagittal, transverse, and frontal images obtained at the level of the tibial tuberosity showing 2 hypoattenuating tracks with normal surrounding bone (*arrowheads*). (B) Frontal and sagittal images obtained at the level of the medial femoral condyle showing a hypoattenuating track extending from the periosteal surface of the medial distal femur to the edge of a cystlike lesion (*arrowheads*). (C) Transverse, frontal, and sagittal images obtained at the level of the medial tibial condyle showing 2 hypoattenuating tracks, of which the most caudal one (*arrowhead*) has a branch extending to the edge of the cystlike lesion (*arrowheads*). On B and C, sclerosis is present around the cystlike lesions and the hypoattenuating tracks. All these tracks are cylindrical and represent vascular channels in normal (A) and pathologic bone (B and C).

- Absence of hypoattenuating line overlying subchondral bone and direct contact of contrast medium with the adjacent subchondral bone, representing full-thickness loss of cartilage
- Accumulation of contrast medium within a subchondral bone defect representing an articular cartilage defect and communication of the subchondral bone defect with the joint

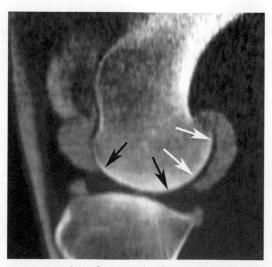

Fig. 7. Sagittal plane reconstruction of a normal stifle CTR. Note the hypoattenuatting interface between the accumulation of contrast medium and the subchondral bone of the medial femoral condyle (*white arrows*). Absence of accumulation of contrast medium is seen between the medial meniscus and the cranial aspect of the medial femoral condyle due to a lack of space between the articular cartilage and the meniscus (*black arrows*).

Unfortunately, evaluation of the weight-bearing articular cartilage of the femoral condyles may not be possible. Despite distension of the joint with contrast medium, there can be inadequate distribution of contrast medium between the menisci and the femoral condyles (see **Fig. 7**). In addition, the menisci are attached to and cover most of the tibial articular surface and do not allow contrast to contact the articular surfaces. In some cases, contrast medium may diffuse into the cartilaginous and/or subchondral bone defects with flexion and extension of the joint following contrast medium administration. In such cases, the abnormal accumulation of contrast medium indicates the presence of an articular cartilage defect. Cases with radiographically questionable communication of an osseous cystlike lesion with the joint space may show evidence of a cartilage defect by accumulating contrast within the cystlike lesion (**Fig. 8**).

Menisci and Meniscal Ligaments

Meniscal lesions
The normal meniscus on CTR should be seen as a uniform filling defect with a semilunar shape on sagittal and frontal reconstructions, and on transverse images they have a "c" or "inverted c" shape curving along the abaxial periarticular margins of each respective tibial condyle (**Fig. 9**).

A meniscal lesion may consist of a tear, prolapse, collapse, or a combination of any of them (**Fig. 10**). Secondary dystrophic mineralization may also be present (**Fig. 11**).

Stifle CTR features of meniscal injuries
- Tears that extend to the surface of the meniscus are evident by diffusion of contrast medium within the substance of the meniscus in a transverse or longitudinal linear or irregular/amorphous fashion
- Contrast outlining the meniscus will reveal abnormalities in size, shape, or position. A prolapse is evident by extension or prominent bulge of the outer margin of

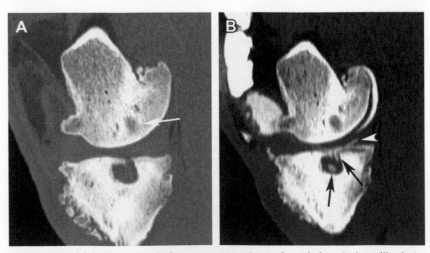

Fig. 8. (*A*) CT and (*B*) CTR sagittal plane reconstructions of a subchondral cystlike lesion of the medial tibial condyle. Note the contrast medium diffusing into the lesion (*black arrows*) through a meniscal tear (*white arrowhead*). There is sclerosis and a noncommunicating subchondral cystlike lesion on the adjacent femoral condyle (*white arrow*). In addition, there is a large amount of sclerosis around the cystlike lesions and irregular periosteal new bone formation and periarticular osteophytes on the proximal tibia and distal femur.

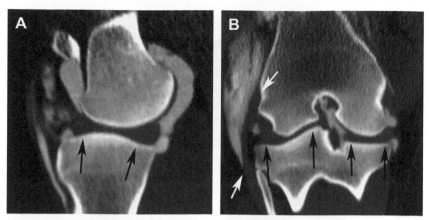

Fig. 9. (*A*) Sagittal and (*B*) frontal plane reconstructions of a normal stifle CTR. Note the "semilunar" shape of the menisci as hypoattenuating structures between the femoral and tibial condyles (*arrows*). There is no evidence of contrast medium diffusion into the meniscal tissue. The arrowheads indicate a normal lateral collateral ligament.

the meniscus beyond the periarticular margins. Abaxial prolapse is more common; however, caudal and potentially cranial prolapse may also occur.
- A collapse is evident by thinning of the hypoattenuating joint space between the adjacent tibial and femoral condyles

Evaluation of the meniscal ligaments
All 5 meniscal ligaments are usually visible with an adequate CTR technique. These ligaments include the cranial and caudal medial meniscotibial ligaments, the lateral cranial and caudal lateral meniscotibial ligaments, and the lateral meniscofemoral ligament. The lateral caudal tibial meniscal ligament is short and thin, making it challenging to evaluate, especially when the ligament is not surrounded by contrast medium.

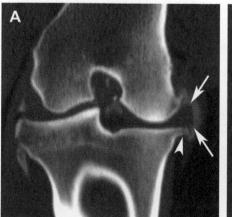
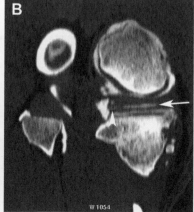

Fig. 10. Frontal plane reconstructions of medial meniscal lesions. (*A*) Marked displacement of the abaxial border of the meniscus (*arrows*) representing a meniscal prolapse. Note the periarticular osteophyte on the abaxial margin of the medial tibial condyle (*arrowhead*). (*B*) Linear (*arrow*) and small multifocal (*arrowhead*) diffusion of contrast medium into the caudal horn of the meniscus (*arrow*) representing a tear.

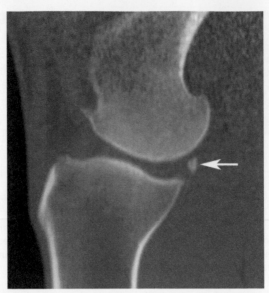

Fig. 11. Sagittal plane reconstruction showing a triangular osseous body with rounded borders in the region of the caudal horn of the medial meniscus (*arrow*) representing dystrophic mineralization.

Tears of the cranial meniscotibial ligaments are more common than damage to the caudal meniscotibial ligaments (**Fig. 12**). Enthesopathy and avulsion fractures may also occur at the insertion sites of these ligaments (**Fig. 13**).

CTR features of meniscal ligament injuries
 • Tears are evident by diffusion of contrast into the body of the ligament in a transverse or longitudinal linear fashion. Multiple linear tears may be present. Irregular contrast diffusion is less common. In addition, enlargement or thinning of the meniscal ligaments may also occur and is identified as contrast outlines the superficial ligament margins.

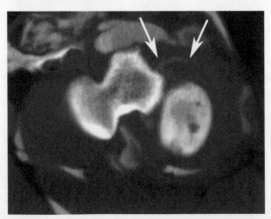

Fig. 12. Transverse plane reconstruction of a cranial medial meniscotibial ligament tear. Note the linear diffusion of contrast medium into the body of the ligament along the longitudinal axis of the fibers (*arrows*).

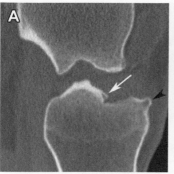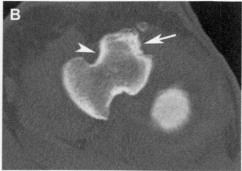

Fig. 13. (*A*) Frontal and (*B*) transverse plane reconstructions showing enthesopathy at the insertion of the cranial medial meniscotibial ligament (*arrows*). Compare with the smooth surface for the insertion of the cranial lateral meniscotibial ligament (*white arrowhead*). A periarticular osteophyte is present on the abaxial margin of the medial tibial condyle (*black arrowhead*).

- Enthesopathy may be evident as an irregular bony surface with bone production, resorption, or a combination of both.
- Small osseous bodies within the ligament and an associated irregular enthesis are highly suggestive of an avulsion fracture.

Cruciate Ligaments

On precontrast images, the cruciate ligaments are difficult to evaluate. However, despite the extracapsular location of the cruciate ligaments, both are visible with an adequate CTR examination. Normal cruciate ligaments on CTR are identified as uniformly hypoattenuating bands of tissue surrounded by contrast medium. Lesions that affect the outer layer or that produce thickening of the ligament, or that break the synovial sheath and allow direct contact of the ligament with the contrast medium, can be identified (**Fig. 14**). Avulsion fractures, enthesopathy, and dystrophic mineralization are also evident with CT.

CTR features of cruciate ligament injuries

- Diffusion of contrast medium into the cruciate ligament from an injury that affects the outer layer of the ligament and subsequently is in contact with contrast medium
- Ligamentous thickening evident by a focal convex outlining of the ligament. This lesion is more difficult to identify and may represent diffuse thickening secondary to inflammation or chronic injury with scar tissue formation.
- Disorganized collection of contrast medium in the region of the cruciate ligament with no evidence of linear outlining of the ligament by contrast medium represents a complete rupture
- Enthesopathy evident by the presence of irregular bony surface with either bone production, bone resorption, or both at the site of enthesis
- Avulsion fractures seen as osseous bodies within the ligament with an associated irregular enthesis

Miscellaneous Soft Tissue Structures

Other soft tissue structures that are visible during CT and CTR include the following: patellar and collateral ligaments, popliteal, common digital extensor, and peroneus tertius tendons (**Fig. 15**). The joint capsule is not commonly seen, although thickening,

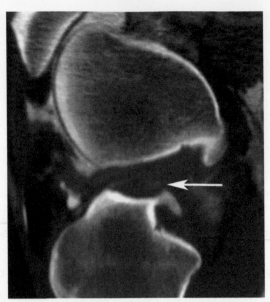

Fig. 14. Sagittal plane reconstruction showing an irregular area of contrast medium diffusion into the distal half of the cranial cruciate ligament (*arrow*) representing a tear.

synovial proliferation, or scar formation of the joint capsule can increase its conspicuity. If proliferative synovitis is present, irregular filling defects may be seen. In cases of severe stifle disease, in which rupture of the joint capsule is present, failure of complete joint distention with leakage and extension of a large amount of contrast

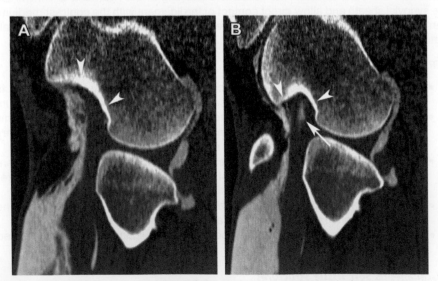

Fig. 15. Sagittal plane reconstructions of the same horse at the level of the extensor fossa (*arrowheads*). (*A*) Normal segment of the peroneus tertius tendon and (*B*) a segment of the same tendon with an irregular area of contrast medium diffusion at the origin (*arrow*) representing a partial tear.

medium along the fascial planes of the musculature adjacent to the tear will be evident (**Fig. 16**). Extravasation of a small amount of contrast medium through the injection site is possible; it will not cause failure of complete joint distention and should not be confused with joint capsule rupture.

ADVANTAGES AND DISADVANTAGES OF STIFLE CTR

The equine stifle joint is a complex anatomic region that often presents diagnostic challenges. Many imaging modalities can be used to investigate lameness originating from the stifle joint. Unfortunately, there is not always a specific imaging protocol or flow chart that follows the lameness examination. A diagnostic imaging approach/plan should be developed between the clinician and the radiologist with the goal of obtaining the most accurate diagnosis for determining an appropriate treatment plan.

Advantages of CTR
- Rapid image acquisition with excellent spatial resolution and ability to perform MPR with unlimited angle orientation
- Excellent image quality for evaluation of all skeletal structures with plain CT
- Diagnosis of cartilage defects and potential joint communication of a subchondral bone lesion
- Diagnosis of meniscal, ligament, and tendon lesions
- Diagnosis of joint capsule tears

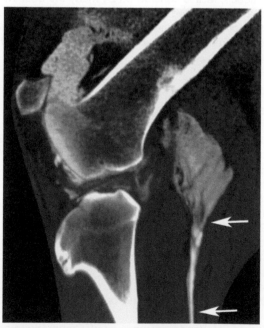

Fig. 16. Sagittal plane reconstruction of a stifle with diffusion of contrast medium between muscle planes on the caudal aspect of the joint (*arrows*) secondary to a joint capsule tear. Despite the extra injection of contrast medium, adequate filling of the stifle joint compartments was not achieved.

Disadvantages of CTR

- Requires general anesthesia
- Usually higher in cost than ultrasound and radiography together
- Potential chance of missing a lesion if abnormal architecture is not present and/ or the lesion is not in communication with the joint space (never in contact with the contrast medium)
- Potential chance for nondiagnostic arthrograms (requires adequate arthrographic technique)
- Potential risk for iatrogenic joint infection as with any kind of arthrocentesis
- Cannot identify osseous fluid that does not have associated structural abnormalities, such as would occur with a contusion
- Inconsistent visibility of surface fraying lesions (cranial tibial meniscal ligament fraying as seen with arthroscopy)
- Articular cartilage intrasubstance abnormalities, such as diffuse degeneration or scar formation, cannot be identified with CTR
- Inadequate visualization of the articular cartilage surfaces of the distal femoral condyles

SUMMARY

CTR is an imaging modality that should be considered an option for the diagnosis of stifle lameness in horses. The clinician should also keep in mind that in many cases the combination of commonly used imaging techniques (radiography and ultrasonography) with or without additional arthroscopic examination does not provide a complete evaluation of all structures that comprise the stifle joint. In human medicine and small animal practice, MRI is considered by many the best imaging modality for diagnosing joint disease. The limited availability of MRI equipment that can adequately image an equine stifle joint, long image acquisition times, and the cost of MRI examinations make CTR an extremely valuable option for the diagnosis of equine stifle joint disease.

REFERENCES

1. Barrett MF, Frisbie DD, McIlwraith CW, et al. The arthroscopic and ultrasonographic boundaries of the equine femorotibial joints. Equine Vet J 2012;44:57–63.
2. Watts AE, Nixon AJ. Comparison of arthroscopic approaches and accessible anatomic structures during arthroscopy of the caudal pouches of equine femorotibial joints. Vet Surg 2006;35:219–26.
3. Baxter GM, Stashak TS. Perineural and intrasynovial anesthesia. In: Baxter GM, editor. Adams & Stashak's lameness in horses. 6th edition. West Sussex (UK): Wiley-Blackwell; 2011. p. 197–9.
4. Bergman EH, Puchalski SM, Veen van der H, et al. Computed tomography and computed tomography arthrography of the equine stifle: technique and preliminary results in 16 clinical cases. Lexington (KY): American Association of Equine Practitioners (AAEP); 2007. p. 46–55.
5. Corbetti F, Malatesta V, Camposampiero A, et al. Knee arthrography: effects of various contrast media and epinephrine on synovial fluid. Radiology 1986;161:195–8.
6. Vekens EV, Bergman EH, Vanderperren K, et al. Computed tomographic anatomy of the equine stifle joint. Am J Vet Res 2011;72:512–21.

The Basics of Musculoskeletal Magnetic Resonance Imaging
Terminology, Imaging Sequences, Image Planes, and Descriptions of Basic Pathologic Change

Matthew D. Winter, DVM, DACVR

KEYWORDS

- Magnetic resonance imaging • Pulse sequences • Imaging planes
- Musculoskeletal imaging

KEY POINTS

- Magnetic resonance (MR) imaging provides unparalleled image contrast and has become instrumental in diagnosing the causes of equine lameness.
- There are multiple types of MR imaging sequences and image planes that allow for improved lesion characterization and more accurate prognosis.
- Understanding the different types of image contrast, including methods of fat suppression, is important in interpreting MR images and in lesion characterization.
- Many, but not all, lesions in the musculoskeletal system manifest as increases in signal intensity.
- Artifacts, when present, must be recognized to ensure that they are not misinterpreted as lesions.
- MR imaging technology is rapidly advancing, and will continue to provide new methods of lesion detection in the future.

INTRODUCTION

Enthusiasm for magnetic resonance (MR) imaging has increased greatly over the last 2 decades and has been motivated by the abundance of information that can be acquired in an MR study. As a cross-sectional imaging modality that uses the inherent magnetic properties of tissue, MR imaging provides exceptional tissue contrast and allows for imaging in multiple slices made through the anatomy of interest. The

Funding sources: None.
Conflicts of interest: None.
Small Animal Clinical Sciences, College of Veterinary Medicine, University of Florida, 2015 SW 16th Avenue, Gainesville, FL 32610, USA
E-mail address: mdwinter@ufl.edu

information obtained is based on the structure and biochemical environment of hydrogen atoms in the tissues. This information can reveal important clinical data regarding lesions and their underlying pathophysiologic mechanisms, especially in the complicated soft tissue structures of the equine distal extremity.

The ability to acquire so much information is of great benefit in the diagnosis of musculoskeletal injury in the equine patient. However, there are many considerations regarding availability, expense, and communication that ultimately affect the usefulness of such a powerful imaging modality. As with any diagnostic imaging technique, the value of the study is directly related to the quality of the image. Image quality can be influenced by several factors, including magnetic field strength, gradient strength, field of view (FOV), image acquisition software, patient preparation and positioning, and operator experience. These features can be generally categorized into equipment-based factors and operator-based factors.

Other variables that affect the usefulness of the MR examination in the equine distal extremity are the choices of area imaged, sequences, and image planes. Lameness localization is often challenging and is of utmost importance because it defines the area to be imaged. Diagnostic imaging is a key component of the lameness examination, and radiography as well as ultrasonography are commonly performed following lameness localization. With radiography and ultrasonography, obtaining additional images of different areas is quick and convenient. In comparison, MR studies are more expensive, require more time to acquire, and can require general anesthesia. Because of these requirements, the number of regions that can be imaged in 1 study is necessarily limited, placing increased importance on lameness localization and sequence selection.

The choice of MR image sequences and planes is based on a desire to provide exceptional image contrast and spatial resolution between normal and abnormal tissues while minimizing the length of the MR examination, especially when the patient is under general anesthesia. These choices are influenced by the signalment, history, and lameness examination findings, and are also based on the knowledge and experience of the imager as the examination progresses.

This article reviews the effects of imaging equipment, image sequences, and image planes on the accuracy of MR imaging of the equine distal extremity and reviews how commonly encountered lesions may alter MR appearances of musculoskeletal anatomy in the equine patient.

Terminology

The terminology pertaining to MR images and pulse sequences can be complicated. Terminology often refers to equipment, imaging sequences, and study planning. A summary of commonly encountered MR terminology is provided here.

- Proton. The MR image is generated from mobile hydrogen atoms, which are often referred to as protons, or spins. Simply put, these polarized atoms containing a single proton and a single electron act as tiny magnets, and moving magnets can generate an electrical signal in a nearby coil of wire. This signal is the basis of MR imaging.
- Magnetic field strength. The main magnetic field is responsible for creating a uniform magnetic environment for the protons to exist in equilibrium. Measured in Tesla (T), greater magnetic field strength generally creates images with better contrast and more signal. The strength of the magnetic field affects the quality of the image, equipment cost, and study cost. Field strength is typically divided into low and high field.

- ○ Low field strength. Low-field magnets generally range from 0.15 T to 0.5 T. Low-field magnets are typically permanent magnets and require less money to purchase and maintain. In addition, resolution is decreased with low-field magnets compared with high-field magnets, and some sequences are limited.
- ○ High field strength. High-field magnets range from 1.0 T to 3.0 T, with MR units of greater field strengths (7 T and beyond) available primarily for research applications. The benefits of high-field magnets include increased speed of image acquisition, increased spatial resolution, and increased FOV.
- FOV. FOV describes the amount or scope of anatomy that is included in a single study. The FOV should encompass the area of concern, but can be limited by the size of the MR unit, the amount of time available for scanning, and the amount of spatial resolution desired in the image. In general, increasing the FOV without changing other imaging parameters increases the amount of signal available from the tissues, but decreases spatial resolution.
- Radiofrequency pulse. As stated earlier, the protons exist in the uniform environment of the main magnetic field. The process of creating signal from the patient involves excitation of those protons, which requires the addition of energy and is accomplished by the use of a radiofrequency pulse that affects the equilibrium of the protons.
- Gradient. In creating the MR image, it is often important to generate small amounts of known variation in the uniformity of the main magnetic field. This variation is achieved by using added coils of wire that can create a range of small magnetic field changes. These changes are referred to simply as gradients, and are an integral part of the MR imaging system. The speed and strength of the gradients in an MR imaging system have a direct effect on the performance of the system and on image quality.
- Signal intensity. This term generally refers to the degree of brightness of a particular tissue in an image. It is common to describe the brightness, or intensity, of a lesion in terms of its signal relative to a normal structure that may be a normal portion of the same structure (ie, the deep digital flexor tendon), or a structure in the vicinity. Signal intensity for the same structure may be different on different sequences.
  - ○ Hyperintense (high signal intensity). Those structures that are bright on an MR image are referred to as hyperintense. This term is also used when a structure is brighter than is normally expected on that specific sequence.
  - ○ Hypointense (low signal intensity). Those structures that are dark on an MR image are referred to as hypointense. This term is also used when a structure has lower signal than is normally expected for that specific tissue on a specific sequence.
  - ○ Isointense. Those structures with the same intensity are referred to as isointense.
  - ○ Intermediate signal intensity. Those structures that are medium gray on an MR image can be referred to as intermediate in signal intensity.
- Signal/noise ratio (SNR). SNR is a quantitative value that is often used generically to refer to the amount of signal that is generated by the tissue versus the amount of signal generated by random events or background noise. Background noise does not provide information about the area being imaged and is detrimental to image quality. If there is more noise than true signal, then image quality is poor. For example, when imaging a fetlock, it is ideal to have the maximum amount of signal generated by the tissues of the fetlock, and a low amount of signal resulting from random radiofrequency events and background noise.

Therefore, the goal of all imaging is the highest possible SNR. SNR increases in a nearly linear relation to magnetic field strength

- Sequence. This term refers to the pattern and timing of specific imaging parameters that define how an image was obtained. This terminology also typically includes information about the type of contrast present in the image (image contrast is discussed later).
  - ○ Spin echo (SE). SE refers to a set of sequences that rely on a series of radio-frequency pulses and applications of gradients to obtain images. These fundamental sequences provide large amounts of signal, and can take long periods of time to acquire.
  - ○ Fast spin echo (FSE). FSE is a modification of the spin echo technique that allows for significant decreases in acquisition time with minimal sacrifices in image quality. Also referred to as turbo spin echo (TSE), this subset of sequences has become the mainstay of most imaging protocols.
    - ■ FSE images can be T1 weighted (T1W), T2 weighted (T2W), or proton density weighted (PDW) depending on imaging parameters.
  - ○ Gradient echo or gradient recalled echo (GRE). These terms refer to a set of sequences that rely on series of gradient applications rather than radiofrequency pulses to create MR images. Gradient echo sequences are typically faster than SE sequences and can provide thinner slices in the same amount of time as an SE sequence. However, the superior spatial resolution of GRE is often offset by the poor contrast/noise ratio achieved with these sequences. In addition, artifacts are more prevalent.
    - ■ GRE images can be T1W, T2W, or a combination of T1W/T2W depending on imaging parameters.
- Image contrast. The goal of any diagnostic imaging is to emphasize visual differences between normal and abnormal tissues. An image with high contrast is typically more black and white, with fewer shades of gray, like painting a picture using only 2 colors. An image with low contrast typically has many shades of gray, and although it may be aesthetically pleasing, like painting a picture with a full palate of colors, the ability to distinguish one type of tissue from another is reduced. Somewhere in between is typically ideal because too few shades of gray can also prevent differentiation of various structures, whereas too many shades of gray can obscure abnormalities. With radiography, and even ultrasonography, the ability to differentiate between normal and abnormal tissue can be limited by the amount of contrast in the image. One of the strengths of MR is that contrast can be created in the image by manipulating the parameters of image acquisition. In general, contrast is described in terms of T1 weighting and T2 weighting, proton density weighting, and T2* weighting. The appearance of these different tissues with different contrast weighting reflects the different physical and magnetic properties of different tissues, and allows separation of fat, fluid, muscle, and tendons/ligaments. An in-depth discussion of these properties is beyond the scope of this article. The interested reader is referred to additional resources for further information.[1–3]
  - ○ T1 weighting. In general, T1 weighting results in an image with high signal intensity and good anatomic detail, but lower contrast in that there tends to be more shades of gray (**Fig. 1**A). Fat is bright (hyperintense), and fluid is dark (hypointense), with muscle having an intermediate (gray) signal intensity between fat and fluid. Cortical bone, tendons, and ligaments appear dark, or hypointense, because of a generally low number of mobile protons.

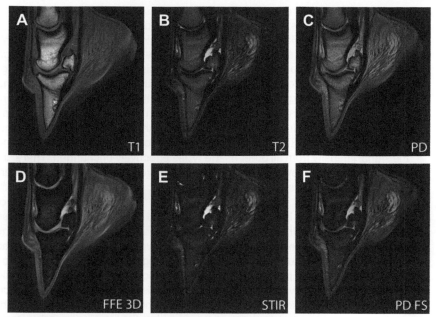

Fig. 1. Sagittal images of the distal extremity of a horse showing the differing contrast characteristics of T1W (*A*), T2W (*B*), PDW (*C*), T2* (*D*), short tau inversion recovery (STIR) (*E*), and proton density (PD) FS (*F*) images. Note the high signal intensity of the trabecular bone reflecting the presence of fat in images on the FSE images (*A–C*), and how this signal is decreased in images that use FS techniques (*D–F*). In addition, note the low signal intensity of the fluid in the distal interphalangeal joint and the navicular bursa on the T1W image (*A*) compared with the other images (*B–F*). In addition, note that there is no signal associated with the hoof wall, and that the signal seen surrounding the distal phalanx represents the laminae. Finally, also notice the more intermediate signal of the soft tissues in the PD FS image (*F*) as compared to the STIR image (*E*).

- ○ T2 weighting. In general, T2W images have lower signal than T1W and PDW images. However, with current technology, T2W FSE images have excellent image quality. In addition, contrast resolution between normal and abnormal tissues is sometimes greater in T2W images than in other SE or FSE images (see **Fig. 1**B). Fat is bright (hyperintense) on FSE/TSE images, fluid is bright (hyperintense), and muscle is of intermediate signal intensity. As with T1W images, cortical bone, tendons, and ligaments appear dark, or hypointense.
- ○ Proton density weighting. Sequences that minimize both T1 and T2 weighting are referred to as PDW, because the signal intensity and the contrast in PDW images are solely related to the concentration of mobile protons in the tissue or organ (see **Fig. 1**C). These images typically have high SNR with hyperintense fluid, intermediate fat, and intermediate muscle. As with other contrast weighting, cortical bone, tendons, and ligaments remain hypointense.
- ○ T2* weighting. In general, T2*-weighted (T2*W; pronounced T2-star) images have contrast characteristics similar to those of T2W images but are created using gradient echo techniques (see **Fig. 1**D). This sequence can typically be acquired more quickly and may allow for thinner slices. However, this sequence is the most susceptible to artifacts caused by differences in magnetic field uniformity and abrupt changes that occur at interfaces with

tissues that have different magnetic properties. As with T1W and T2W images, cortical bone, tendons, and ligaments remain hypointense.

○ Fat suppression (FS). In considering the descriptions of T1W, T2W, and PDW imaging earlier, it may seem confusing and counterintuitive that fat retains high signal intensity with each type of contrast weighting. It has already been suggested that many lesions tend to have increased signal intensity in MR, and separating the high signal intensity from fat and the high signal intensity from an abnormality becomes important in evaluation of an MR image. One way that contrast is most frequently manipulated in an effort to isolate high signal intensity lesions in MR imaging is by elimination of the fat signal while leaving the signal intensity from all other tissue types effectively unchanged. There are multiple ways to achieve this goal; 2 that are more commonly used are inversion recovery and fat saturation.

  ▪ Inversion recovery. This technique is based on the known behavior of fat-bound protons in a strong magnetic field and manipulation of these protons such that they are unable to generate a signal in the image. The high signal generated by fat is reversed, or inverted, through the use of an additional radiofrequency pulse into the imaging sequence. For suppression of fat, this inversion pulse arrives early in the sequence, and is therefore said to require a short inversion time. As a result, this is often referred to as short tau (or time) inversion recovery (STIR) sequence (see **Fig. 1E**). This technique can be used at both low-field and high-field imaging, and is most commonly used with T2 or PD weighting. In addition, the elimination of the fat signal from a sequence with a long repetition time (TR) and echo time (TE) often results in an image with low SNR and poor spatial resolution. This spatial resolution is sacrificed for the gains in contrast resolution and benefits to lesion characterization.

  ▪ Fat saturation (FS). This technique is based on the ability of the MR unit to know what signal is coming from protons located in fat as opposed to protons located in water, and negate any signal from the protons in fat (see **Fig. 1**F). This technique can be applied to T2W, PDW, and T1W images. Achieving sufficient fat saturation can be challenging, and the success of this technique depends on magnetic field strength, the uniformity of the magnetic field, and the proximity of material with different magnetic properties. In addition, this technique is not possible with low-field magnets and is best achieved at 1.5 T and higher field strengths.

• Resolution. Resolution commonly refers to the ability to distinguish 2 (or more) objects from one another. In diagnostic imaging, contrast resolution and spatial resolution are often referred to in relation to image quality and diagnostic value.

○ Contrast resolution refers to the ability to distinguish 2 (or more) structures based on differences in their signal intensity on an image. MR has high contrast resolution compared with radiography, computed tomography (CT) or ultrasonography. SE and FSE sequences have higher contrast resolution than GRE sequences.

○ Spatial resolution refers to the ability of the imaging system to resolve 2 (or more) objects that are close to one another, but are still separate. Spatial resolution in MR is dictated by field strength, gradient strength, and other imaging parameters such as matrix size and slice thickness. Radiography and CT have greater spatial resolution than MR. GRE sequences have the highest resolution relative to acquisition time and achieve this by a sacrifice in contrast resolution.

- Image plane. Because MR imaging is a cross-sectional imaging modality that has the ability to create thin slices of anatomy, slice positioning should be carefully considered. With MR, images can be made in a nearly infinite number of planes, but typically are created in 3 orthogonal planes: transverse, sagittal, and dorsal (**Fig. 2**). It is useful to have slices that are perpendicular to the area of interest (an articular surface, for example). It is also important to confirm the presence of a lesion on more than 1 imaging plane. The definitions below relate specifically to imaging of the appendicular skeleton, but can be extrapolated to the axial skeleton as needed.
  - Sagittal plane. A vertical plane parallel to the long axis of the bone that divides the limb into medial and lateral parts (see **Fig. 2A**).
  - Dorsal/frontal/coronal plane. These terms are often used interchangeably, and indicate a plane that is parallel to the long axis of the bone that divides the limb into dorsal/cranial and palmar/plantar/caudal parts (see **Fig. 2B**).
  - Transverse/axial plane. These terms are often used interchangeably, and indicate an image plane that is perpendicular to the long axis of the bone, dividing regions into proximal and distal (see **Fig. 2C**).

To summarize the use of these terms, the sequence and imaging plane are typically described, followed by the anatomic location, affected structure, and signal intensity when describing abnormalities. Using the definitions of MR terminology discussed earlier, an example of a typical MR imaging sequence of the fetlock might be referred to as SAG T2 FSE, which would indicate a series of slices made in a medial-to-lateral plane, oriented parallel to the long axis of the distal extremity, with T2 weighting, and obtained using a FSE (or turbo spin echo image) technique. Another imaging sequence that might be encountered is DOR PD FSE FS, which describes a series of slices made from dorsal to palmar/plantar, oriented parallel to the long axis of the bones, using a PDW FSE technique with added fat saturation. Taking this a step further, a description of the abnormality might include high signal intensity in the medial condyle of the third metacarpal bone on the DOR PD FSE FS sequence, indicating the presence of fluid.

Equipment

The generation of an MR image is based on the movement of hydrogen atoms, or protons, in the body. These mobile protons act as miniature magnets that can generate a measurable electrical current. The basic components of MR imaging are mobile protons in the body, a strong magnetic field, magnetic gradients,

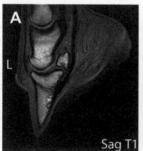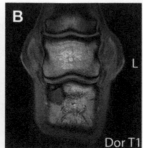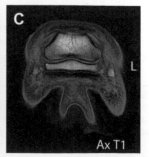

Fig. 2. Sagittal (*A*), dorsal (*B*), and transverse/axial (*C*) T1W images of the left distal extremity of a horse. There is a round, well-defined, hypointense lesion in the medial aspect of the distal phalanx that would be better characterized with additional sequences (see **Fig. 3**).

radiofrequency waves to add energy to the protons to make them move, and a receiver coil that collects the electrical signal generated by the moving protons. A computer with acquisition software is needed to time these events and generate an image from the electrical signals.[2,3]

Imaging Sequences and Tissue Appearance

As stated earlier, the MR image is based on the movement of protons in the body. The amount of proton movement depends on the environment of protons, specifically their chemical bonds in the tissues. The tissue environment of a proton therefore affects the amount of signal it can generate, and the relative brightness of that tissue on an image. Alterations in the expected signal intensities for a given tissue help identify specific types of lesions in that tissue, such as increased fluid signal in bone, changes in ligament and/or tendon signal patterns, and/or soft tissue injury. Different sequences provide different tissue contrast, and it is the summation of the information acquired in each sequence and each plane that allows for more accurate diagnosis and prognosis in cases of equine lameness.

Relative brightness or darkness of a tissue also depends on the imaging sequence that is performed (see **Fig. 1**). The most fundamental pulse sequences are T1W, T2W, and PDW sequences. Knowing the typical appearances of general tissue types, such as fat, muscle, tendon, and fluid, can aid in the identification of abnormal signal characteristics, because pathologic change that alters regional environments manifests on an MR image as alterations in expected signal intensity.

Sequences are generally described in terms of the imaging parameters that dictate the time between radiofrequency pulses (TR) and the time at which the signal is collected (TE). The amount of T1, T2, or PD weighting in an image is a function of the chosen TR and TE (**Table 1**).

Sequence Selection

Maximizing contrast differences that occur because of pathologic change is directly related to the choice of pulse sequence. A steady stream of new pulse sequences is constantly being introduced, resulting in new ways of manipulating image contrast. The choices can be overwhelming and confusing, therefore a review of commonly applied sequences is necessary to understand MR examinations. Findings on each type of sequence must be evaluated to reach a more complete understanding of the pathologic change present.

PDW images have excellent resolution and tissue contrast with clear delineation between synovial fluid and joint capsule as well as articular cartilage. T2W sequences also provide good tissue contrast, and provide good separation of fluid, soft tissue, and fat signals.

T1W sequences provide excellent anatomic detail. However, the contrast between soft tissue and fluid structures, specifically between synovial fluid and the joint capsule, is less than is possible with PDW and T2W images. T1W images are

Table 1		
Table of repetition times (TR) and echo times (TE) that determine contrast weighting on standard spin echo images. These values are different on GRE images, in which weighting is also related to other sequence parameters, such as flip angle, which are not discussed here		
	Short TR (<800 ms)	**Long TR (>2000 ms)**
Short TE (<40 ms)	T1 weighted	Proton density weighted
Long TE (>60 ms)	Not typically used	T2 weighted

commonly used for evaluation of contrast enhancement characteristics associated with infection, inflammation, or neoplasia such as keratoma, although postcontrast imaging has been performed with PDW sequences.

FS techniques are of utmost importance in establishing delineation between fluid signal that may represent a true lesion and surrounding, normal fat. STIR images, PD FS images, or T2 FS images should be compared with PDW or T2W images, preferably in the same imaging plane. STIR images are good for use in low-field systems, in which fat saturation sequences are not possible.[2] In addition, STIR works well with large FOV imaging, in which the magnetic field inhomogeneities may cause inconsistent FS using chemical shift–based techniques.[2] In addition, STIR may be the best option to rule out incomplete fat saturation that may occur in the location of susceptibility artifacts[2] caused by residual rust in the hoof wall from shoeing nails. Fat saturation techniques are almost always better than STIR images at high field because of increased SNR, and can be applied to T1W, T2W, and PDW sequences as well.

An imaging protocol or series of different sequences is typically grouped together to image a patient. A musculoskeletal protocol typically includes a T2, PDW, PDW FS, and STIR. Including both FS and STIR images allows for a more robust distinction between fat and fluid. On PD FS images, fat saturation can occasionally be incomplete, and including STIR images can help confirm areas of true fluid accumulation. PD FS images tend to have a greater SNR, with better image quality compared with a STIR image.

Image Area and Imaging Planes

The patient's clinical signs define the imaging area, and the importance of a thorough lameness evaluation cannot be overemphasized. In addition, the size of the imaging area varies based on magnet type, and the image FOV has direct effects on image resolution and SNR. It is not possible to easily image numerous areas efficiently without compromising image quality and even patient safety, because prolonged lateral recumbency can potentially result in severe myopathy.

In general, our defined imaging regions for MR imaging studies of the distal extremity are similar to those used for radiography. We image the foot and distal pastern, the fetlock and proximal pastern, the high suspensory, or the carpus/tarsus. Stifle MR imaging can be performed in selected cases, depending on magnet design and horse conformation. In addition, studies of the head and the cranial cervical spine may be performed in some magnets with appropriate bore diameter and coil availability.

Usefulness of Multiple Sequences

The imaging sequences are designed to reveal the signal intensity of different tissues in a predictable fashion, therefore alteration of the signal intensity in tissue on different sequences can reveal detailed information about lesion content and severity (**Figs. 3 and 4**). It is important to recognize that the same tissue can have similar signal intensity on certain sequences. Examples include fluid and sclerosis, which cannot be distinguished on a T1W image, and fat and fluid, which cannot be distinguished on a T2W image. Therefore multiple sequences must be used in conjunction to accurately characterize a lesion.

How to Find Abnormalities on MR Studies Based on the Report Description

As mentioned earlier, most MR imaging protocols are made up of a combination of sequences that are designed to maximize identification of all types of abnormalities. A well-designed protocol includes multiple sequences, including some form of FS, and multiple imaging planes. Most abnormalities can be identified on PDW or T1W

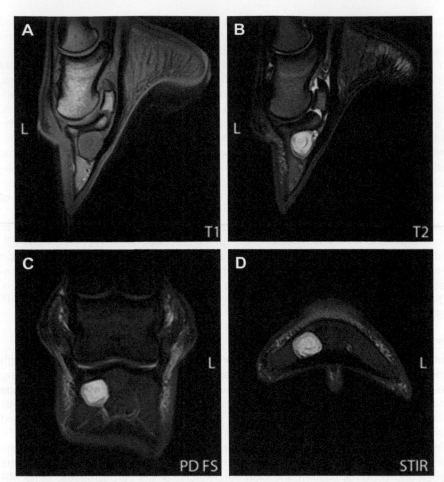

Fig. 3. Sagittal T1W image (*A*), sagittal T2W image (*B*), dorsal PDW image (*C*), transverse/axial STIR image (*D*), and parasagittal gross pathologic section (*E*) of the left (*L*) distal extremity of a horse with a round, well-defined, T2-hyperintense lesion in the medial aspect of the distal phalanx. Note the high signal of this lesion on the T2W, PDW, and STIR images and low signal on the T1W image. In addition, the lesion has a nonuniform, swirling appearance and passes through the palmar cortex of the distal phalanx. The lesion is indicated by an asterisk (*) in (*E*). There was firm, gelatinous material in this lesion on gross examination. Although the signal intensity of this lesion appears similar to the signal intensity of fluid, it is several shades of gray darker on the PDW and T2 images and has mixed signal intensity. The impression that it has a high fluid content is correct. However, this signal pattern, which is several shades of gray darker and of mixed signal intensity, on these sequences is significant and important to recognize. It shows the difference between pure fluid and more solid, gelatinous material, as was present in this case.

sequences. Fluid signal often correlates with severity, so evaluating the same area on T2W and fat-suppressed images yields additional information regarding the severity of the lesion. Selecting the correct imaging plane also makes identifying the abnormality easier. Finding an abnormality on multiple imaging planes is the key to knowing it is real. A lesion typically is most easily identified on 1 or 2 planes, and may be more difficult to identify on the third plane.

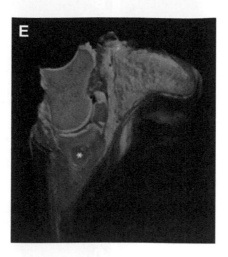

Fig. 3. (*continued*)

In general, imaging planes that are perpendicular to the structure being evaluated are best for characterizing changes. This generalization is commonly true for soft tissue structures of the distal extremity that run parallel to the long axis of the limb, including the collateral ligaments, sesamoidean ligaments, and the flexor and extensor tendons (**Figs. 5** and **6**). For this reason, it becomes necessary to plan imaging planes carefully, because small changes in imaging plane angle can increase the sensitivity of the imaging study. However, even when positioning the limb with the toe pointed, small changes in planning the transverse imaging plane may be required to obtain transverse images of the deep digital flexor tendon at the level of the navicular bone and insertion on the palmar cortex of the distal phalanx. The length of a tendon or ligament lesion may be best determined on another orthogonal plane. For the soft tissues located dorsal and palmar/plantar to the distal extremity, the transverse plane best shows the lesion. However, the sagittal plane is often best for assessing lesion length.

Evaluation of cartilage and subchondral bone is made more complex by the curvature of the articular surfaces. Curved surfaces have increased artifact that can obscure margins, making it more difficult to accurately identify articular cartilage lesions. Articular surface lesions are often best seen on sagittal and dorsal planes. However, those articular lesions located at the extreme dorsal or extreme palmar/plantar aspect of joints, particularly in the fetlock, may be best seen on transverse image planes because the transverse plane is perpendicular to the most dorsal and palmar articular surfaces. Because identification of a lesion on more than 1 imaging plane is generally required to confirm its presence, slight alterations in planning the angle of orthogonal images may be required to definitively identify a lesion on the second plane. As an example, oblique frontal planes are often performed in the fetlock positioned as perpendicular as possible to the dorsodistal and dorsopalmar surfaces of the condyles because of high incidence of disease in these regions and reduction in artifact as result of the change in slice positioning.

Identification of Pathologic Change

One of the greatest strengths of MR imaging is its ability to identify changes in fluid content in tissue. In general, inflammatory and neoplastic processes result in the recruitment of cells, hemorrhage, and edema to the affected region. This increased

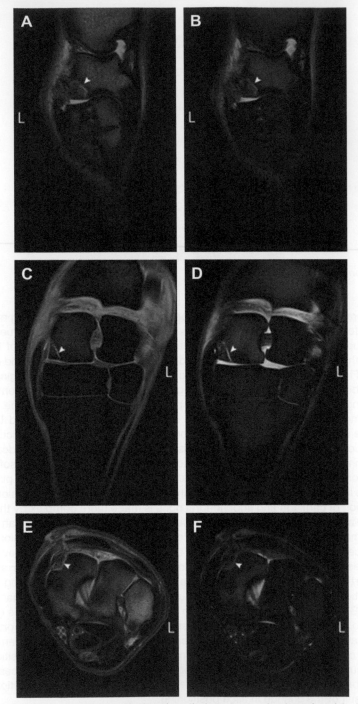

Fig. 4. Sagittal PDW (*A*) PDW FS (*B*), dorsal spoiled gradient echo (SPGR) FS (*C*), dorsal PDW FS (*D*), transverse PDW (*E*), and transverse STIR (*F*) images of the left carpus of a horse with an arthroscopically created fracture of the dorsodistomedial aspect of the left carpus (*arrowhead*). Note the increased signal intensity localized to the radiocarpal bone on the fat-suppressed images. Also note the thickening and increased signal intensity in the dorso-medial soft tissues as well as effusion associated with recent arthroscopy.

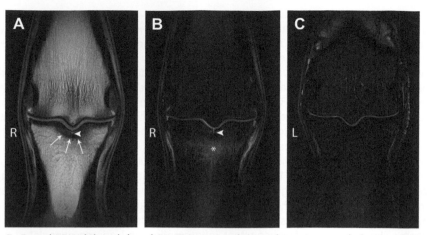

Fig. 5. Dorsal PDW (*A*) and dorsal PD FS images of the right metacarpophalangeal joint of a horse with an incomplete sagittal fracture of the right proximal phalanx (*arrowhead*). A PDW FS image with normal bone signal of the left metacarpophalangeal joint (*C*) is provided for comparison. Note that the linear hyperintensity (*arrowhead*) representing the fracture on the PDW and PDW FS images is surrounded by a relatively hypointense region suggesting sclerosis (*arrows*). On the PDW FS image (*B*), note the region of ill-defined increased signal intensity (*asterisk*) that is not seen on the image of the normal left metacarpophalangeal joint.

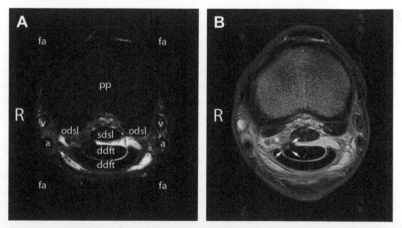

Fig. 6. Transverse STIR (*A*) and transverse PDW (*B*) images of a right pastern obtained at the level of midproximal phalanx. Note the high-signal-intensity lesion (*arrows*) and deformation of the lateral lobe of the deep digital flexor tendon (ddft). This high signal intensity persists on the STIR image, although it is less hyperintense. In addition, note the presence of hypointense material located between the deep digital flexor lesion, the lateral oblique distal sesamoidean ligament (odsl), and the straight distal sesamoidean ligament (sdsl). a, proper palmar digital artery; ddft, deep digital flexor tendon; fa, flow artifact; odsl, oblique distal sesamoidean ligament; pp, proximal phalanx; sdft, superficial digital flexor tendon; sdsl, straight distal sesamoidean ligament; v, proper palmar digital vein.

fluid associated with inflammation is most easily identified on STIR images or on PD and T2 images with fat saturation (see **Fig. 4**B). Over time, particularly in soft tissues, as the process resolves and the fluid decreases, the increased signal in these abnormal tissues gradually resolves.

Fibrosis also causes significant changes in relaxation times and therefore alters the expected signal intensities in a given tissue. As mentioned earlier, mobile protons are a necessary component in MR imaging. Fibrous tissue in general contains few, if any, mobile protons, and therefore provides little signal on MR images. However, early fibrosis has slightly higher signal on T2W images, whereas the signal associated with mature fibrosis is significantly reduced.[4]

The presence of fat in muscles and other musculoskeletal tissues produces a predictably high signal on T1W and T2W images as discussed earlier. Hemorrhage also causes a variety of changes in expected tissue signal intensity; changes depend primarily on the location of the hemorrhage and its stage of degradation. Acute or subacute hemorrhage in muscle or other tissues tends to cause increased signal intensity, likely because of concomitant inflammation and edema associated with the underlying cause. However, collections of blood such as hematomas have a variable appearance on MR images based on the age or duration of the process because of the formation of paramagnetic substances as the iron in each erythrocyte is oxidized and ultimately exposed to surrounding water molecules. Hemorrhage degradation byproducts may remain in the tissues for an extended period of time and may have associated abnormal signal intensity.

Alterations in bone signal can represent a variety of changes. One of the most commonly described changes in bone reflects an increase in bone signal intensity on STIR, PD FS, and T2W FSE/TSE images (fluid sensitive sequences), and a decrease in signal intensity on T1W images (see **Figs. 3** and **4**). This change is often specifically referred to as a bone marrow edema pattern, bone bruise, or bone contusion. Depending on the distribution, the term occult fracture is also sometimes used to describe these findings. These terms can be misleading, in that these MR findings result from a multitude of pathologic processes that may not be distinguished from one another on MR imaging. In addition, this finding can correlate with histopathologically diagnosed bone edema. However, other causes for increased bone signal intensity pattern include bone marrow fat necrosis, abnormal trabeculae, bone marrow fibrosis, subchondral pseudocysts, bone marrow bleeding, microfractures in various stages of healing, and normal bone marrow elements.[5–7] It is therefore more appropriate to refer to these lesions as bone marrow lesions or high-signal-intensity bone lesions.[8]

Alterations in the trabecular bone pattern can be seen with high-field MR imaging.[9] Recent histologic correlation with fat-suppressed MR images of the navicular bone depicting increased bone signal intensity showed a combination of changes including fat atrophy, with lipocytes showing loss of definition of cytoplasmic borders, a proliferation of capillaries within the altered marrow fat, perivascular or interstitial edema, enlarged intertrabecular bone spaces, fibroplasia, and thinned trabeculae showing loss of bone.[10]

Other studies have identified the extension of increased bone signal intensity lesions on STIR or PD FS images into the subchondral bone plate.[11] This finding correlated with lameness in all reported cases. However, resolution of lameness does not always correlate with a resolution of increased bone signal intensity on STIR images. It has been reported in horses and in people that increased bone signal intensity can persist on STIR images despite resolution of lameness or pain.[8,12–15] More recently it has been reported that persistently increased bone signal intensity in the navicular bone is associated with chronic lameness.[10] Therefore, the persistence of increased bone signal intensity and its relationship to continued lameness may depend on anatomic location and the specific bone affected.

Subchondral bone plate thickness has not been described for each joint of the equine distal extremity, but, in the tarsus, certain patterns have been described that generally reflect loading stress.[16] Asymmetric changes in subchondral bone plate thickness can reflect modeling of the subchondral bone, often referred to as subchondral bone plate thickening. However, delineation between cartilage and subchondral bone, and delineation between subchondral bone and cancellous bone, can be challenging.[17] The accuracy of this distinction is influenced by the choice of imaging sequence. It has been reported that this delineation is best made on MR imaging using GRE FS and spoiled gradient echo (SPGR) or SPGR FS sequences.[17]

Evaluation of cartilage thickness in normal horses and the detection of cartilage lesions have been studied.[17–21] Complete assessment of cartilage thickness, erosions, or tears is not routinely possible using radiography or ultrasonography, and MR techniques are particularly well suited for cartilage evaluation. Accurate assessment of articular cartilage is made challenging by the curvature of the articular surfaces in the distal extremity as well as the thin layer of articular cartilage present, especially in the metacarpophalangeal and metatarsophalangeal joints. As before, the availability of at least 1 orthogonal plane increases the likelihood of an accurate diagnosis, and this is also true of cartilage lesions.[18] Sequences that have been used for this assessment include T2*W GRE and T1W SPGR (T1 SPGR) and SPGR with FS (T1 SPGR FS) techniques.[17,18,21–23] These sequences have been reported to provide excellent delineation between cartilage and subchondral bone margins. In general, mensuration of cartilage thickness on MR images is overestimated, but MR measurements have been shown to correlate with histomorphometric measurements in the carpus using SPGR images.[17]

The literature suggests that imaging cartilage at low field does not yield significant information regarding the integrity of articular cartilage.[23] However, in 1 study, evaluation of the distal interphalangeal joint using a low-field system did allow the identification of large, partial-thickness erosions using high-resolution T1W GRE images.[18] However, in that study, superficial, partial-thickness cartilage irregularities were not identified using any sequence in any plane.[18] Cartilaginous lesions have also been reported to be more accurately represented using PD FS and T2 sequences.[23]

At high-field imaging, the agreement between histologic measurement of cartilage and measurements made on T1W SPGR FS images has a good correlation,[21] and the FSE/TSE images are most accurate in delineating the size and shape of detected cartilage lesions in an experimental model.[23] However, even at high-field imaging, experimental cartilage lesions can be difficult to detect, specifically partial thickness lesions. Thin, linear, full-thickness or partial-thickness cartilage lesions are not always identified, and, in general, the severity of cartilage damage can be underestimated.[21,23] In experimental models, additional findings that might support cartilage injury are not present. The effect of concomitant changes in subchondral bone signal intensity and the presence of bone marrow lesions in the region of cartilage injury have not been assessed by these studies.

The evaluation of ligaments and tendons with MR, especially in areas of the distal extremity that are less accessible with ultrasound, has been reported to be a more sensitive, specific, and accurate method of examination compared with ultrasound, with greater reproducibility.[24] Normal ligaments and tendons generally have low signal intensity and appear hypointense on all sequences because of their lack of mobile protons. Significant lesions associated with ligaments and tendons typically involve edema, increased cellularity, and occasionally hemorrhage, and can manifest as increased signal intensity on T2W and PDW images (see **Fig. 5**).[4] Lesion distribution depends on the tendon or ligament being considered. For example, lesions in the deep digital flexor tendon vary in their location (dorsal abrasion, core lesion, parasagittal split) depending on the level of the lesion (ie, at the level of the distal impar sesamoidean ligament, the navicular bone, the collateral sesamoidean ligament, the navicular bursa, or the distal interphalangeal joint).[25] In addition, signal changes in tendons and ligaments that are contoured or curved may show increased signal intensity resulting from magic angle artifact.[26–29] Magic angle artifact occurs in sequences with low TE values when the fibers of a tendon or ligament are oriented at approximately 55° to the main magnetic field.[3] The resultant increased signal intensity may be misinterpreted as a lesion, which commonly occurs at the distal aspect of the deep digital flexor tendon and may also occur in the collateral ligaments. Resolving tendon and ligament lesions are characterized by a progressive reduction in cellularity, edema, and hemorrhage, and manifest on MR images with progressive reduction in signal intensity as the fibrous tissue associated with healing becomes mature.[4]

SUMMARY

The usefulness of MR imaging in the diagnosis of equine lameness is unquestionable. As with most imaging modalities, advances in technology happen very quickly, and the information that can be obtained can seem limitless and overwhelming. A basic understanding of MR sequences, expected signal intensity of normal tissues, and the role of multiplanar imaging is the foundation for interpreting MR images. Although limitations exist, the rapidity with which new techniques and sequences are being developed and the potential for biochemical changes to be indirectly assessed using MR spectroscopy offer possibilities for the continued development of this modality and ensure its continued application in the diagnosis of equine lameness.

REFERENCES

1. Bushberg JT. The essential physics of medical imaging. Philadelphia: Lippincott Williams & Wilkins; 2002.
2. McRobbie DW, Moore EA, Graves MJ, et al. MRI from picture to proton. 2nd edition. Cambridge: Cambridge University Press; 2007.
3. Mitchell D, Cohen M, Cohen M. MRI principles. 2nd edition. Philadelphia: Saunders; 2003.
4. Crass JR, Genovese RL, Render JA, et al. Magnetic resonance, ultrasound and histopathologic correlation of acute and healing equine tendon injuries. Vet Radiol Ultrasound 1992;33(4):206–16.
5. Taljanovic MS, Graham AR, Benjamin JB, et al. Bone marrow edema pattern in advanced hip osteoarthritis: quantitative assessment with magnetic resonance imaging and correlation with clinical examination, radiographic findings, and histopathology. Skeletal Radiol 2008;37(5):423–31.
6. Zanetti M, Bruder E, Romero J, et al. Bone marrow edema pattern in osteoarthritic knees: correlation between MR imaging and histologic findings. Radiology 2000; 215(3):835–40.
7. Zani DD, Zani D, Biggi M, et al. Use of magnetic resonance imaging in the diagnosis of bone marrow edema in the equine distal limb: six cases. Vet Res Commun 2009;33(Suppl 1):225–8.

8. Olive J, Mair TS, Charles B. Use of standing low-field magnetic resonance imaging to diagnose middle phalanx bone marrow lesions in horses. Equine Vet Educ 2009;21(3):116–23.
9. Link TM, Majumdar S, Augat P, et al. In vivo high resolution MRI of the calcaneus: differences in trabecular structure in osteoporosis patients. J Bone Miner Res 1998;13(7):1175–82.
10. Dyson S, Blunden T, Murray R. Comparison between magnetic resonance imaging and histological findings in the navicular bone of horses with foot pain. Equine Vet J 2012. Available at: http://www.ncbi.nlm.nih.gov/pubmed/22494146. Accessed May 1, 2012.
11. Zubrod CJ, Schneider RK, Tucker RL, et al. Use of magnetic resonance imaging for identifying subchondral bone damage in horses: 11 cases (1999-2003). J Am Vet Med Assoc 2004;224(3):411–8.
12. Link TM, Steinbach LS, Ghosh S, et al. Osteoarthritis: MR imaging findings in different stages of disease and correlation with clinical findings. Radiology 2003;226(2):373–81.
13. Holowinski M, Judy C, Saveraid T, et al. Resolution of lesions on STIR images is associated with improved lameness status in horses. Vet Radiol Ultrasound 2010; 51(5):479–84.
14. Dyson S, Nagy A, Murray R. Clinical and diagnostic imaging findings in horses with subchondral bone trauma of the sagittal groove of the proximal phalanx. Vet Radiol Ultrasound 2011;52(6):596–604.
15. Dyson SJ, Murray R, Schramme MC. Lameness associated with foot pain: results of magnetic resonance imaging in 199 horses (January 2001–December 2003) and response to treatment. Equine Vet J 2005;37(2):113–21.
16. Branch MV, Murray RC, Dyson SJ, et al. Is there a characteristic distal tarsal subchondral bone plate thickness pattern in horses with no history of hindlimb lameness? Equine Vet J 2005;37(5):450–5.
17. Murray RC, Branch MV, Tranquille C, et al. Validation of magnetic resonance imaging for measurement of equine articular cartilage and subchondral bone thickness. Am J Vet Res 2005;66(11):1999–2005.
18. Olive J. Distal interphalangeal articular cartilage assessment using low-field magnetic resonance imaging. Vet Radiol Ultrasound 2010;51(3):259–66.
19. Schramme M, Kerekes Z, Hunter S, et al. Improved identification of the palmar fibrocartilage of the navicular bone with saline magnetic resonance bursography. Vet Radiol Ultrasound 2009;50(6):606–14.
20. Smith MA, Dyson SJ, Murray RC. Reliability of high- and low-field magnetic resonance imaging systems for detection of cartilage and bone lesions in the equine cadaver fetlock. Equine Vet J 2012. Available at: http://www.ncbi.nlm.nih.gov/pubmed/22435499. Accessed May 1, 2012.
21. Olive J, D'Anjou MA, Girard C, et al. Fat-suppressed spoiled gradient-recalled imaging of equine metacarpophalangeal articular cartilage. Vet Radiol Ultrasound 2010. Available at: http://doi.wiley.com/10.1111/j.1740-8261.2009.01633.x. Accessed May 2, 2012.
22. Smith MA, Dyson SJ, Murray RC. Reliability of high- and low-field magnetic resonance imaging systems for detection of cartilage and bone lesions in the equine cadaver fetlock. Equine Vet J 2012. Available at: http://www.ncbi.nlm.nih.gov/pubmed/22435499. Accessed May 20, 2012.
23. Werpy NM, Ho CP, Pease AP, et al. The effect of sequence selection and field strength on detection of osteochondral defects in the metacarpophalangeal joint. Vet Radiol Ultrasound 2011;52(2):154–60.

24. Rand T, Bindeus T, Alton K, et al. Low-field magnetic resonance imaging (0.2 T) of tendons with sonographic and histologic correlation. Cadaveric study. Invest Radiol 1998;33(8):433–8.
25. Dyson S, Murray R. Magnetic resonance imaging evaluation of 264 horses with foot pain: the podotrochlear apparatus, deep digital flexor tendon and collateral ligaments of the distal interphalangeal joint. Equine Vet J 2007;39(4):340–3.
26. Spriet M, Zwingenberger A. Influence of the position of the foot on MRI signal in the deep digital flexor tendon and collateral ligaments of the distal interphalangeal joint in the standing horse. Equine Vet J 2009;41(5):498–503.
27. Spriet M, McKnight A. Characterization of the magic angle effect in the equine deep digital flexor tendon using a low-field magnetic resonance system. Vet Radiol Ultrasound 2009;50(1):32–6.
28. Smith MA, Dyson SJ, Murray RC. Is a magic angle effect observed in the collateral ligaments of the distal interphalangeal joint or the oblique sesamoidean ligaments during standing magnetic resonance imaging? Vet Radiol Ultrasound 2008;49(6):509–15.
29. Werpy NM, Ho CP, Kawcak CE. Magic angle effect in normal collateral ligaments of the distal interphalangeal joint in horses imaged with a high-field magnetic resonance imaging system. Vet Radiol Ultrasound 2010;51(1):2–10.

Use of Intravenous Gadolinium Contrast in Equine Magnetic Resonance Imaging

Travis C. Saveraid, DVM[a],*, Carter E. Judy, DVM[b]

KEYWORDS

- Equine • Magnetic resonance imaging • Gadolinium • Contrast
- Contrast-enhanced MRI

KEY POINTS

- Gadolinium contrast-enhanced magnetic resonance imaging (MRI) is an easily performed add-on procedure in equine MR studies that can improve lesion detection.
- Contrast-enhanced MRI provides additional anatomic and physiologic assessment of pathologic change beyond standard MR sequences.
- To allow for direct comparison of precontrast and postcontrast images, including performing subtraction, all precontrast and postcontrast images need to be acquired before moving the patient. Subtraction images should be interpreted with caution because the signal patterns on these images have not been validated in the equine patient, and any associated artifacts are not fully known.

INTRODUCTION

Despite the clinical use of equine magnetic resonance imaging (MRI) for nearly 15 years, gadolinium-based contrast-enhanced MRI (CE-MRI) is performed very uncommonly and is rarely reported.[1–6] In people, MR contrast is used routinely in central nervous system, oncologic, infectious, and angiographic and perfusion imaging studies.[7] MR contrast is also commonly used in small animal imaging, for primarily the same applications including neurologic, oncologic, and vascular imaging.[8] In horses, the use of gadolinium contrast imaging has been reported, often as an aside, in case reports and small clinical series in brain, laryngeal, and septic arthritis studies.[1–4] The authors' group has published and presented several small studies and early initial experiences with equine orthopedic CE-MRI.[5,6,9]

The authors have nothing to disclose.
[a] VetRadiologist LLC, 1776 Wellesley Avenue, St Paul, MN 55105, USA; [b] Alamo Pintado Equine Medical Center, 2501 Santa Barbara Avenue, PO Box 249, Los Olivos, CA 93441, USA
* Corresponding author.
E-mail address: travis@vetradiologist.com

DEVELOPMENT OF INTRAVENOUS MRI CONTRAST DOSE

In 2007, the authors began to administer intravenous MR contrast during equine musculoskeletal imaging examinations to see if lesion conspicuity would increase. At that time there was no information in the literature regarding a favorable dose for contrast in equine MRI studies. The only reference to contrast enhancement was a total dose of 20 mL/adult horse of gadodiamide (Omniscan; GE Healthcare, Waukesha, WI) administered intravenously during equine brain studies at Washington State University College of Veterinary Medicine.[1] This dose was chosen originally by necessity, as only one 20-mL vial of contrast was available in the hospital when the first equine brain study was performed (Pat Gavin, Pullman, WA, personal communication, 2003).

Six gadolinium-based contrast agents (GBCA) are approved by the US Food and Drug Administration (FDA) for use in the central nervous system.[10] This group of agents is used most commonly in general veterinary imaging. The approved contrast dose for 5 of the 6 FDA-approved gadolinium agents is approximately 0.1 mmol/kg or 0.2 mL/kg. Gadobutrol (Gadavist; Bayer Healthcare) is recently FDA-approved, the recommended dose being 0.1 mL/kg (medication package inserts). The 0.2 mL/kg dose is equal to 0.9 mL/10 lb (4.5 kg) or roughly 1 mL/10 lb of gadopentate dimeglumine (Magnevist; Bayer Healthcare, Shawnee Mission, KS) contrast. In the average horse of 1000 lb (453.6 kg), a full standard dose is therefore approximately 100 mL. To test this dosage in the horse, 100 mL of intravenous gadopentate dimeglumine was administered to several cases at Alamo Pintado Equine Medical Center during high-field MRI. The initial assessment was favorable and an in-hospital, prospective study was undertaken to develop an appropriate dose for intravenous gadopentate dimeglumine. Patients in 20 consecutive clinical imaging examinations were injected with contrast at escalating doses. All horses were imaged in a 1.5-T MR system (Siemens Espree; Siemens Medical Solutions USA, Inc, Malvern, PA). The contrast was administered following completion of the standard sequences. Intravenous gadopentate dimeglumine (25 mL) was administered followed by a 1-minute delay, then a T1-weighted volume-interpolated breathhold examination (VIBE) sequence in the axial plane was performed over approximately 3 minutes. An additional 25 mL of intravenous gadolinium contrast was then administered with repeat imaging of the same axial sequence, followed by administration of 50 mL of intravenous contrast with a third repetition of the axial sequence. The precontrast images and the 3 sets of postcontrast images were subjectively and objectively assessed for degree of contrast enhancement of a variety of tissue structures including discovered lesions. The subjective assessment was determined by consensus review by a board-certified radiologist and board-certified surgeon (T.S. and C.J.). Although objective assessment of signal intensity using regions of interest showed a statistically significant difference in contrast versus baseline for all identified lesions, there was a difference in conspicuity of lesions between doses. A full dose of 100 mL/horse provided the most contrast enhancement of tissues, particularly of abnormalities; however, the 50-mL/horse dose resulted in the same subjective lesion conspicuity. The 25-mL/horse dose occasionally failed to show visually obvious contrast enhancement. It was concluded that 50 mL/horse of gadopentate dimeglumine was the most appropriate dose for clinical scanning.

Since that time intravenous contrast enhancement has been used frequently in the equine MRI studies at Alamo Pintado Equine Medical Center. The hospital equine population comes from a variety of performance disciplines including racing Thoroughbreds, high-level eventing Warmbloods, barrel-racing Quarter Horses, and backyard trail horses. As of late 2011, approximately 600 horses have been administered contrast in addition to the routine high-field MRI study. The purpose of this article is to highlight experiences using GBCA in equine MRI. The authors believe that CE-MRI improves the recognition and assessment of the lesions, and aids in guiding further treatments and prognostication.

MR CONTRAST AGENTS

There are currently 8 FDA-approved GBCA MRI agents.[10] However, 2 of the newer agents, gadofosveset trisodium (Ablavar; Lantheus Medical Imaging, North Billerica, MA) and gadoxetate disodium (Eovist; Bayer Healthcare) are specialty agents approved for assessment of the specific disorders aortic iliac disease (gadofosveset trisodium) and focal liver disease (gadoxetate disodium). The other 6 contrast agents are more routinely used in general systemic imaging studies (**Table 1**).

Mechanism of Action of Gadolinium-Based Contrast Agents

Traditional iodine or barium contrast agents used in radiography and computed tomography (CT) are detected because they directly attenuate x-ray photons. MR contrast agents are detected indirectly because of the effects of the gadolinium molecules on the adjacent tissues. Specifically, gadolinium shortens the magnetic relaxation time constants of water in the tissues. The majority of gadolinium contrast applications are focused on imaging the effects of the decreased T1 relaxation time. Shortening of the T1 constant (shortened T1 relaxation time) results in increased signal intensity from enhanced tissues when imaged with short retention time (TR), T1-weighted images.[11]

Unbound gadolinium ion is a heavy metal and, similar to most heavy metals, is a known toxin. However, gadolinium ions used in contrast agents are chelated, resulting in a relatively biologically inert molecule. Chelation of gadolinium ion blocks the cellular uptake of the gadolinium, thus shielding cells from toxic effects. Because the chelated ions are not incorporated intracellularly, gadolinium molecules distributed from the vascular space into the capillaries remain extracellular within the interstitial space.[11] The distribution half-life (the distribution from the vascular space into the interstitial regions) is approximately between 2.5 and 5.0 minutes.[12] The biological half-life of gadolinium products is approximately 1.5 to 2.0 hours.[11]

Possible Adverse Reactions

In general, gadolinium contrast agents are considered safe and have lower incidence rates of reactions than traditional iodinated radiography and CT contrast agents. In

Table 1
Name and basic properties of FDA-approved gadolinium-based contrast agents[a]

Brand Name, Chemical Name	Ionicity	Clearance	Osmolality (mOsm/kg)
Magnevist (gadopentetate dimeglumine, Gd-DTPA	Ionic	Renal	1960
Multihance (gadobenate dimeglumine, Gd-BOPTA)	Ionic	Renal (96%) Hepatic (4%)	1970
Gadavist (gadobutrol)	Ionic	Renal	1603
OptiMARK (gadoversetamide, Gd-DTPA-BMEA)	Nonionic	Renal	1110
Omniscan (gadodiamide, Gd-DTPA-BMA)	Nonionic	Renal	789
ProHance (gadoteridol, Gd-HP-DO3A)	Nonionic	Renal	630

[a] Information from product package inserts.

human studies, most adverse reactions are minor and include headache, injection-site discomfort, and dizziness. The most prominent cardiovascular affect is a transient mild drop in systemic pressure, usually following rapid injection at increased contrast dose rates (greater than typical 0.1 mmol/kg approved dose).[11] Although several of the gadolinium agents have a higher than normal physiologic osmolality, the small total volumes of contrast injected create only a very small increase in transient vascular osmolality, much lower than the osmolality changes seen with iodinated contrast agents for systemic CT imaging.[11] MR contrast agents are considered nonnephrotoxic. However, in people nephrogenic systemic fibrosis (NSF) is a severe, but rare, side effect. NSF occurs in patients with preexisting renal disease who are given intravenous gadolinium-based contrast MRI. NSF results in fibrotic changes within the skin as well as other body organs such as the heart, liver, lungs, and skeletal muscles.[13] NSF has not been documented in veterinary patients.

At the authors' hospital, all patients have preanesthetic screening including complete blood count/serum chemistry panels. Horses are maintained under general anesthesia with isoflurane. Heart rate, direct and indirect arterial blood pressure, O_2 saturation, inspired and expired CO_2, inspired and expired isoflurane, and temperature are recorded and monitored by horse-side staff. The first 2 cases of cranial imaging had a transient drop in blood pressure immediately following the contrast administration. The ultimate reason for the transient decrease in blood pressure was never determined, but this has not reoccurred over the last 50 head cases. No other adverse intrastudy or poststudy effects related to contrast administration have been documented.

PREIMAGING PLANNING
Case Indications for Contrast Use

Use of contrast is typically made on a case-by-case basis, and frequently the decision to administer contrast occurs during the examination based on preliminary assessment of the images (**Boxes 1** and **2**).

Advantages and Potential Drawbacks of Contrast Use

The advantages of using MR contrast, particularly in musculoskeletal imaging, are still being learned and evaluated. The drawbacks have been limited. The initial experiences suggest the advantages and drawbacks listed in **Boxes 3** and **4**.

MR CONTRAST IMAGING TECHNIQUE

- The anatomic region is imaged using routine MRI sequences and positioning.
- T1-weighted images are acquired precontrast.
- Fifty milliliters of gadopentate dimeglumine are administered intravenously via jugular catheter.

Box 1
Indications to use or recommend MR contrast

- All brain studies and most nasosinal studies
- In cases with soft tissue, intracapsular or articular abnormalities, especially lesions of the tendons, ligaments, and subchondral bone identified in the initial standard sequences
- In cases with other unexplained soft tissue or bone lesions
- For most thorough study with owner consent

Box 2
Indications for elective MR contrast use

- Obvious lesions, particularly multiple severe lesions (ie, complete deep digital flexor tendon ruptures), whereby pragmatic clinical judgment suggests that further defining the severity of the lesions is unnecessary
- No lesions identified on the initial standard study

- Sixty seconds is timed before commencing postcontrast T1-weighted sequence acquisition.
- T1-weighted sequences are obtained postcontrast following 60-second postinjection delay.
- The precontrast and postcontrast T1-weighted sequence positioning is identical to allow for digital subtraction images after acquisition.

Imaging Tips
- The authors use T1-weighted VIBE sequences in axial (with fat saturation) and dorsal planes (non–fat saturation); this is a 3-dimensional volume, spoiled gradient echo sequence with echo time (TE) of 3.2 milliseconds, TR of 9.3 milliseconds, and typically a 2-mm image thickness. This sequence has the following advantages:
  o Thin image slices, including submillimeter isotropic, if desired
  o Excellent definition of bone margins and subchondral bone/trabecular bone interface (non–fat saturation)
  o Shorter acquisition times than traditional spin-echo T1-weighted sequences
  o As a T1-weighted gradient echo sequence with a very short TE (3.2 milliseconds), the effects of gadolinium contrast are more conspicuous than spin-echo T1-weighted sequences with longer TE (typically 12–18 milliseconds)[14]
- Postprocessing subtraction images allow for rapid and easier assessment for areas of enhancement.

INTERPRETATION OF CLINICAL CASES
Contrast Enhancement in Normal Anatomy

Morphologic anatomy of the equine limbs in MR images has been well described in previous publications.[15,16] With contrast imaging, the clinician needs to be aware of the normal vascular anatomy and blood distribution. Any structure with a rich blood supply will have visual enhancement. Conversely, relatively avascular structures

---

Box 3
Primary advantages of CE-MRI in horses

- Increased lesion conspicuity
- Potential assessment of active, chronic active, or healed lesion
- Assessment of vascularized or nonvascularized regions
- Potential localization of continued active, abnormal regions within a larger lesion to guide interventional therapy (ie, stem cell therapy in tendon lesions)

Box 4
Potential drawbacks of MR contrast use

- Added cost: The wholesale cost of a 50-mL Magnevist dose is currently $230. The authors purchase 100-mL multiuse vials.

- Longer image acquisition time: Each postcontrast sequence requires 2 to 3 minutes on a high-field magnet; this would likely be longer with low-field systems. Subtraction images are created as a postprocessing step. and this does require additional imaging time.

- Potential for adverse contrast reaction: This factor has not been a problem at the authors' institution.

---

such as normal tendon or cortical bone will not visually enhance (**Fig. 1**). In the limbs, tissues that routinely enhance include vessels, the synovial membranes, and capillary-rich areas of the hoof wall such as the parietal corium and vascular lamina (**Fig. 2**). Noticeably enhancing structures in the head besides normal vasculature include the choroid plexus in the lateral, third, and fourth ventricles, the nasal mucosa, lymph nodes, and salivary glands (**Fig. 3**).

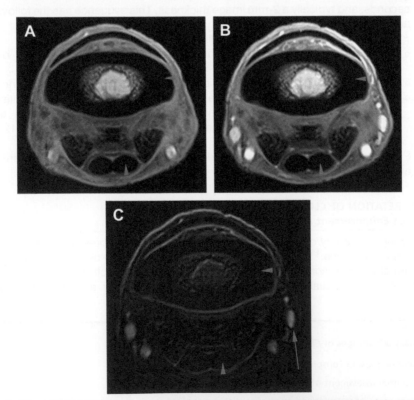

Fig. 1. T1-weighted VIBE axial at the mid level of P1. Images are noncontrast (*A*), postcontrast (*B*), and subtraction (*C*). The arrowheads show the absence of contrast enhancement in the deep digital flexor tendon and the cortical bone. On the subtraction image, contrast enhancement of the palmar digital vessels (palmar vein is indicated by arrow) is apparent.

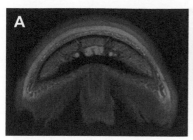

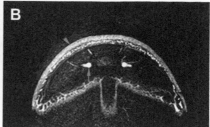

Fig. 2. T1-weighted VIBE postcontrast (*A*) and subtraction (*B*) axial images at the distal portion of P3. The arrowhead shows the marked contrast enhancement of the lamellar layer. Contrast enhancement is also present in the venous terminal arch (*arrow*).

Clinical Uses and Case Examples

Tendons/ligaments

The authors' group has described CE-MRI in tendon and ligament injuries previously.[5,6,9] However, there are no other known publications regarding the use of MR contrast in assessing tendon injuries in horses. The use of contrast-enhanced CT (CE-CT) has been described in evaluating tendon lesions and other lesions in the foot.[17,18]

In CE-MRI, the normal tendon and ligament fascicles have no visible increase in signal intensity. The endotenon connective tissue will have faint contrast enhancement when closely scrutinized (**Fig. 4**). Vascular structures that perforate the tendon or adjacent synovial and paratenon structures are contrast enhanced. With a tendon tear, the orderly tendon fiber pattern is disrupted resulting in disorganized fiber arrangement, increased interstitial space, and altered vascular permeability. The acute inflammatory phase and subacute reparative phase of tendon healing lead to angiogenesis with increased neovascularization, changed vascular permeability, and formation of granulation tissue.[17,19,20]

The specific mechanism for MR contrast enhancement in tendon and ligament lesions is unknown. Within minutes following intravenous injection, the majority of the intravascular contrast distributes into the extracellular, interstitial matrix.[21] Regions of increased vascularity, such as capillary beds and granulation tissue, would

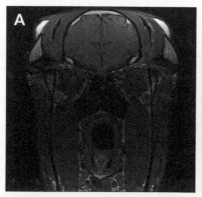

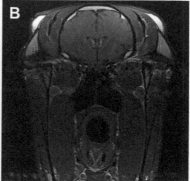

Fig. 3. T1-weighted turbo spin-echo precontrast (*A*) and postcontrast (*B*) images at the mid level of the lateral ventricles. The bilateral choroid plexus of the lateral ventricles has normal robust enhancement, as expected with highly vascularized structures.

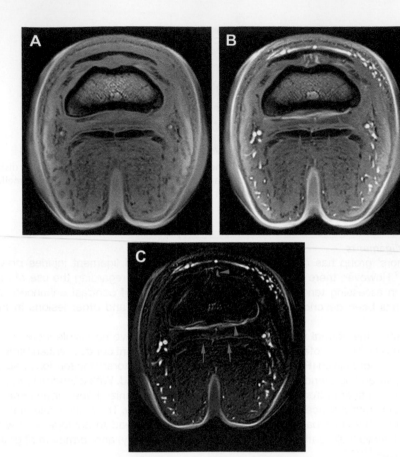

Fig. 4. T1-weighted VIBE precontrast (*A*), postcontrast (*B*), and subtraction (*C*) images of the foot at the level of mid P2 and the proximal aspect of the navicular bursa. The arrows depict the faint contrast enhancement, visible on subtraction images only, of the fine, linear endo-tenon tissue that frequently occurs in normal tendons. The arrowheads indicate areas of mild synovial lining enhancement of unknown clinical consequence in the dorsal proximal and palmar proximal regions of the distal interphalangeal joint.

be expected to have early increased enhancement. In the acute and subacute repar-ative phases of tendon tears, it is speculated that the increased vascularity, vascular permeability, and heterogeneity of the tendon interstitial matrix may allow for greater distribution and persistence of gadolinium molecules within the lesion.[22]

Differentiating the contrast-enhancement pattern between an acute tendon tear and a chronic tear with reoccurring acute injury may not be possible. It is not clear if the contrast enhancement is associated solely with the neovascularization and/or presumed increased vascular permeability with acute tendon tears. Alternatively, contrast enhancement in chronic tears may be the result of chronic alterations in vascular permeability and tendon matrix in the area of reparation. However, similar to previous work,[22] on serial MR examinations the majority of patients with contrast-enhancing lesions on T1-weighted VIBE images have static or increased lameness scores, whereas the majority of patients with lesions that have decreasing contrast enhancement or no enhancement exhibit reduced or absent lameness.

Patients with decreasing or absent signal intensity on the more fluid-sensitive sequences such as T2-weighted and short-tau inversion recovery (STIR) may have improvement in lameness grades or clinical symptoms.[23] T1-weighted images, particularly gradient echo derived sequences, will have persistent signal changes in the lesions for a greater time than the fluid-sensitive sequences.[24] The majority of lesions identified by the authors that have areas of high signal on fluid-sensitive sequences also contrast enhance, suggesting acute tendon injury or active, subacute reparative phase (**Fig. 5**). If the lesion is present primarily on proton-density (PD) and T1-weighted images, but does not contrast enhance, it is assumed that the severity of the lesion is less and the nonenhancing regions of the tendon have remodeled and "healed" (**Fig. 6**). However, occasionally contrast enhancement will occur in a tendon lesion that is only visible on T1-weighted VIBE precontrast and postcontrast images (**Fig. 7**). It is unknown why these lesions show such marked contrast enhancement while remaining essentially normal on other sequences including PD, T2-weighted, and STIR. In these infrequent cases, the lesion seems correlated to the lameness, as no other abnormalities are identified in the imaging examination. While these observations support using contrast-enhancement patterns to assess physiologic "activity" of tendon lesions, it is still fundamentally unknown what causes the clinical "pain" described or identified in human and equine patients with tendon injuries.[25] It remains possible that contrast-enhancement patterns or even signal-intensity patterns on nonenhanced MR sequences may be showing physiologic characteristics of the tendon lesion matrix that are unrelated to the reason for the patient's discomfort.

Lesions within the dorsal margin of the deep digital flexor tendon in the region of the navicular bursa or at the periphery of the superficial or deep digital flexor tendons within the tendon sheath may have additional factors influencing contrast enhancement. The contrast enhancement of dorsal margin lesions may be more noticeable because of the increased neovascularization and recruitment of blood vessels from the subsynovial lining of the navicular bursa, as well as proliferation of granulation tissue (see **Fig. 5**).[17]

Subtraction images of the collateral ligaments of the distal interphalangeal joint are helpful for lesion assessment. These ligaments are particularly susceptible to magic-angle artifact.[26–28] Subtraction images should only show new areas of high signal on T1-weighted images following contrast and remove (make dark) areas of similar signal on the precontrast and postcontrast images, thus negating the confounding high signal from magic-angle artifact. Enhancement still occurs in the regional vessels and fascial planes around and within the ligament, so areas of high signal on subtraction images still require cautious interpretation.

Accurate interpretation of lesions in the distal sesamoidean impar ligament (DSIL) can be challenging, especially when concurrent distal interphalangeal joint synovitis is present. The synovial lining invaginates into the DSIL and if enhancing, the synovitis will mimic or obscure ligament lesions. Coincidental abnormalities such as hyperintensity on STIR images at the osseous attachment sites of the DSIL may support the veracity a DSIL lesion, but interpretation of DSIL disease should still be made with caution.

Synovium

Synovial inflammation and, consequently, contrast enhancement of synovial tissue can occur for several potential reasons such as noninfectious inflammatory arthroses, septic arthritis, and post–intra-articular steroid injection reaction.[4,29,30] Determining the importance of the severity of contrast enhancement is difficult.

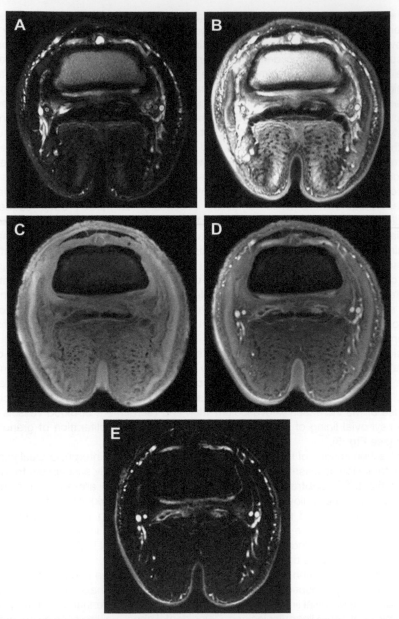

Fig. 5. Axial images mid level of P2 and proximal portion of the navicular bursa. Lameness is localized to the foot region. Extensive areas of tendon fiber disruptions are present in the dorsal half of the medial and lateral deep digital flexor tendon bundles. The lesions have varying degrees of internal hyperintensity on T2-weighted (*A*), proton-density (PD) (*B*), T1-weighted VIBE precontrast (*C*), and T1-weighted VIBE postcontrast (*D*) images. The overlying navicular bursa has thickened walls and is filled with poorly defined proliferative tissue. The subtraction image (*E*) indicates marked contrast enhancement of the tears in the medial and lateral deep digital flexor tendon lobes as well as the enhancement of the bursal lining. Findings are consistent with "active" navicular bursitis and deep digital flexor tendinopathy.

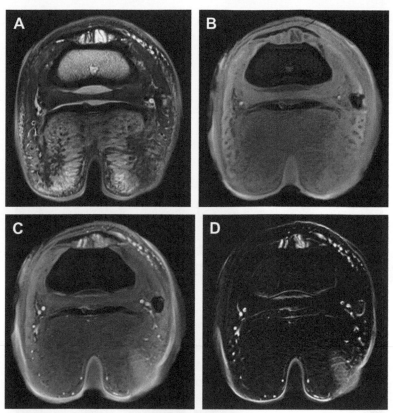

Fig. 6. Axial images mid level of P2 and proximal portion of the navicular bursa. Lameness is localized to the foot region. There is a central, dorsal margin tear of the deep digital flexor tendon. The lesion has increased signal relative to the intact surrounding tendon body on PD (*A*), T1-weighted VIBE precontrast (*B*), and T1-weighted VIBE postcontrast (*C*) images. On the subtraction image (*D*), only the overlying bursa wall or dorsal margin of the tendon enhances, whereas the deeper portion of the lesion does not enhance, suggesting a more quiescent state in the tendon than initially expected.

Marked contrast enhancement of the synovial lining and proliferative synovium has been identified in cases of septic arthritis. The presence of intracapsular, non–contrast-enhancing tissue aggregates are likely fibrin, associated with the marked inflammatory response.[4] Additional findings in confirmed cases of septic arthritis include subchondral bone sequestrum formation, spiderweb-like hyperintensity within the deeper trabecular bone, and capsular and pericapsular enhancement.[4] Variable contrast enhancement and synovial thickening are also seen in noninfectious, inflammatory arthroses (**Fig. 8**). One must keep in mind that contrast enhancement of the synovium may be reduced following intra-articular therapies such as steroid injection.[31]

Occasionally the synovial lining will not have noticeable enhancement. However, it is more common to see patients with mild contrast enhancement of the synovial lining with or without joint effusion (**Fig. 9**). Whether this is a reflection of contrast enhancement of normal synovium or indicates a mild but clinically relevant synovitis is difficult to determine, particularly if there are no other demonstrable lesions in the

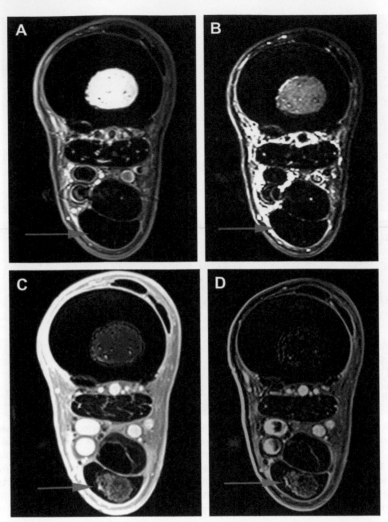

Fig. 7. Axial images from the mid level of the third metacarpal region from a horse with grade 2/5 lameness localized to above the metacarpophalangeal joint region. The *arrows* depict the area of interest in the superficial digital flexor tendon. There are no noticeable abnormalities on the PD (*A*) or short-tau inversion recovery (STIR) (*B*) images. On T1-weighted VIBE postcontrast (*C*) and subtraction (*D*) images, a large central area of contrast enhancement is present in the superficial digital flexor. Given the lack of other abnormal imaging findings, the superficial digital flexor lesion was presumed to be associated with or responsible for the clinical lameness.

imaged region. In people with rheumatoid arthritis, the rapidity and severity of contrast enhancement of the synovium can be correlated with histologic evidence of active inflammation.[32] In the authors' experience, horses with mild synovial enhancement but no other abnormalities in the joint space often have more severe lesions, such as a deep digital flexor tendon tear, in an anatomic separate location, suggesting that the mild synovial enhancement is an incidental or less important finding.

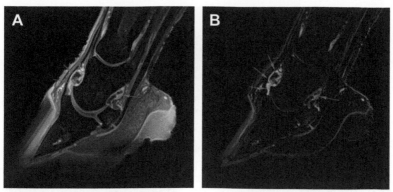

Fig. 8. Sagittal postcontrast (*A*) and subtraction (*B*) images of a case of distal interphalangeal joint synovitis. The synovial tissues of the distal interphalangeal joint are thickened and markedly contrast enhancing (*arrows*). The arrowhead highlights additional contrast enhancement in the palmar aspect of the navicular bone.

As mentioned previously, over time contrast diffuses across the synovium, resulting in blurring of the synovial margins and lack of visual separation of the synovium and the joint fluid. Because of the intracapsular diffusion, the synovial structures should be imaged within 10 minutes after contrast enhancement.[33]

Tendon sheath
CE-MRI has been reported in people to allow for earlier diagnosis of tenosynovitis because of increased recognition of inflammatory changes in the synovial lining of the tendon sheath.[29] In the authors' opinion, contrast allows for greater confidence

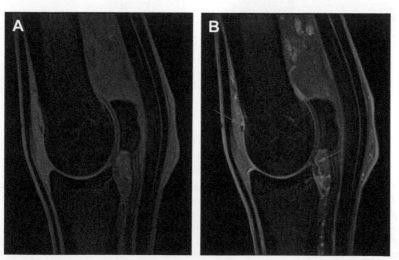

Fig. 9. Sagittal precontrast (*A*) and postcontrast (*B*) images of a metacarpophalangeal joint diagnosed as normal on the imaging study. The thin, but contrast-enhancing synovial lining of the joint capsule, is visible (*arrows*). The joint is not effusive. The articular, subchondral, and periarticular regions of the joint were normal on the rest of the study. A proximal suspensory lesion diagnosed on more proximal MRI (not shown) was presumed to be associated with the grade 2/5 lameness.

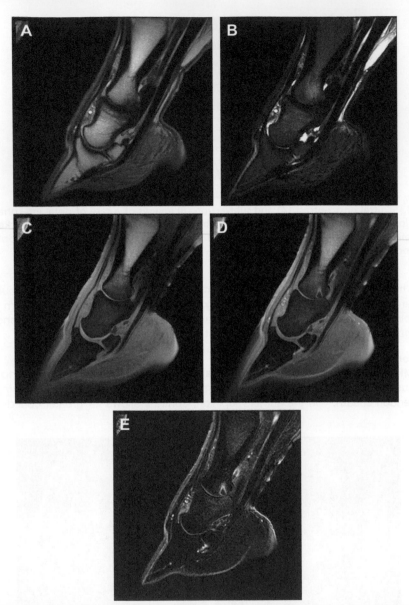

Fig. 10. Sagittal images of distal P1 subchondral bone lesion. A wedge-shaped low-signal region is present in distal P1 subchondral bone region on PD (*A*), STIR (*B*), T1-weighted VIBE precontrast (*C*), and T1-weighted VIBE postcontrast (*D*). A thin rim of high signal surrounds the wedge-shaped low-signal region. Extensive regional high (fluid) signal is also present on the STIR throughout distal P1. The postcontrast and subtraction (*E*) images increase the conspicuity of affected region and depict the difference in the tissue matrix along the peripheral portion of this lesion, as compared with the surrounding trabecular bone and central area.

in diagnosing the severity or activity of the tenosynovitis in the flexor tendon sheath, and may improve detection of margin tears of the deep digital flexor tendon or superficial digital flexor tendon, particularly in the proximal phalangeal region.

Bone

Contrast enhancement does occur in bone, including the subchondral bone and deeper trabecular regions. Subchondral cysts actively enhance, usually along the periphery or lining of the cyst (**Fig. 10**). Trabecular and subchondral contrast enhancement is often present in a location similar to that of the "bone edema" signal on fat-suppressed images. The medullary enhancement may be associated with the similar mechanisms of bone marrow remodeling that result in increased signal on fat-suppressed images; namely, the replacement of the normal marrow matrix in conjunction with increased vascular permeability and angiogenesis. In humans and guinea

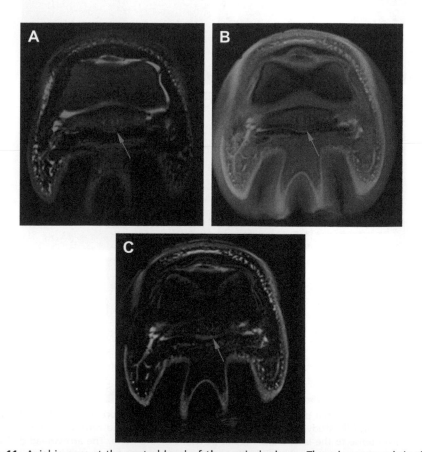

Fig. 11. Axial images at the central level of the navicular bone. There is a very subtle thin line of high signal on the STIR image (*A*) along the central, palmar surface of the flexor cortex of the navicular bone (*arrow*). This line was not recognized on initial review. After contrast (*B*) and subtraction (*C*) images, the contrast enhancement at the same location (*arrow*) suggests an erosive lesion of the flexor cortex or the dorsal surface of the deep digital flexor tendon. Bursoscopy identified an adhesion between the dorsal margin of the deep digital flexor tendon and the flexor cortex of the navicular bone and granulation type tissue filling the flexor cortex erosion.

pigs, contrast-enhancement perfusion studies of bone have been used to estimate contrast outflow ("washout") in subchondral bone edema lesions. Delay in contrast outflow is speculated to indirectly indicate increased intraosseous pressure, which is considered a cause of patient pain in bone edema lesions.[34] This technique may allow for improved evaluation and guide therapeutic decisions in similar lesions of horses.

Contrast enhancement is frequently used in imaging of small joints in the hands, wrist, and foot for assessments of various immune-mediated arthritides and

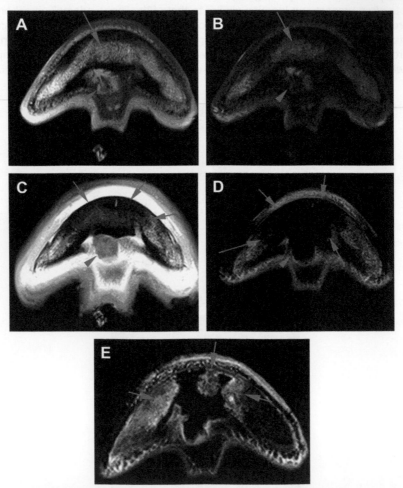

Fig. 12. This patient had unknown penetrating solar trauma approximately 10 to 14 days before the first MRI study. On the initial axial PD image (*A*), the central portion (*arrow*) of P3 is isointense to the lateral and medial portions of the bone. The arrowhead denotes a mixed signal intensity pocket of fluid. Trabecular bone hyperintensity consistent with fluid or "bone edema" is present on the STIR (*B*) image. T1-weighted VIBE postcontrast (*C*) and subtraction (*D*) images revealed a surprising massive void of enhancement consistent with bone infarction in the central portion of the bone (*arrows*). Three weeks later (subtraction image, *E*) the zone of infarction had already decreased in size, presumably secondary to re-establishment of blood supply to the peripheral portions of the affected zone. The STIR images at the 3-week point were nearly identical to the original STIR images, even though there was progressive change on the contrast-enhanced images.

infections.[35–37] Contrast enhancement allows for improved recognition of bone edema and subtle cortical erosion as well as early detection of synovial and tenosynovial enhancement.[32,33] Similarly, contrast enhancement is useful in detecting subtle erosive lesions of the flexor cortex of the navicular bone (**Fig. 11**).

The absence of contrast enhancement is also helpful in assessing for ischemic regions of bone. The absence of enhancement within a larger region of inflammatory change can indicate broad regional infarction or sequestra secondary to severe bone trauma or osteomyelitis. The ischemic areas can appear similar to the surrounding bone, especially in the acute phases of the lesion (**Fig. 12**).

Hoofwall and laminar tissues
Contrast enhancement within the corium parietis and inner lamellar layer is prominent, as is expected for these richly vascular regions. For unexplained reasons, contrast will often be absent in large regions of the lamella and corium (**Fig. 13**), which is specu-lated to be secondary to vasoconstriction during anesthesia or from limb positioning. When this occurs, it is typically in either the lateral or medial aspect of the hoof, not both, but does not appear to be affected by limb positioning because the region can be on either side of the foot. The effect is apparent on multiple sequences throughout the course of the study. With close evaluation of the hoof structures, similar areas of decreased vascular signal can be appreciated on T2-weighted and STIR images, but the large regional absences of blood flow are more noticeable, and confirmed following contrast injection. The authors have not documented later development of laminitis in these feet. When the affected feet are reimaged as part of follow-up for other lesions, the previously affected regions will often be normally enhancing. Dynamic CE-CT evaluation of the hoof wall and laminar structures has been described.[35] Potentially CE-MRI may be useful in future research and clinical evaluation of laminar vascular dynamics.

Head
Contrast enhancement of the tissues of the head is similar to that in canine and feline MRI. Postcontrast T1-weighted images are acquired in 1 to 3 planes in canine and

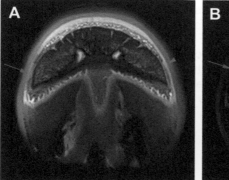
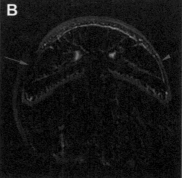

Fig. 13. T1-weighted VIBE axial postcontrast (*A*) and subtraction (*B*) images of the foot at the distal level of P3. Note the regional absence of contrast enhancement in the lamellar and corium parietis (*arrow*) versus the normal enhancement of these structures on the opposite side of the hoof wall (*arrowhead*). The etiology of the nonenhancement is unknown, but may derive from transient vasoconstriction, vascular obstruction or, less likely, positional flow dynamics.

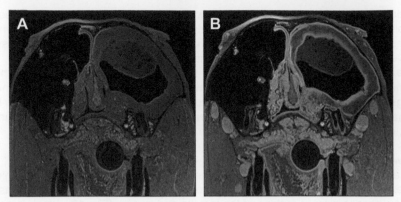

Fig. 14. T1-weighted VIBE axial precontrast (A) and postcontrast (B) images of a horse with previous treatment for sinusitis. A thick rim of contrast-enhancing soft tissue fills the right caudal maxillary and conchofrontal sinuses. Histopathology of the proliferative peripheral zone of tissue indicated chronic granulation tissue.

feline brain and head imaging protocols. The reasons to use contrast in equine head imaging are similar to those regarding small animals, including defining areas of inflammatory change in soft tissues or bone, regions of breakdown of the blood-brain barrier, and improved anatomic definition of masses. Lesions in the brain or spinal cord (which can usually only be included in studies of foals) on standard imaging sequences should be followed with additional postcontrast images to gain the best information for evaluation. Equine brain MR studies for nonspecific, suspected neurologic disease, such as "headshaking," have been unrewarding. Contrast images have been helpful in assessing dental and sinus disease. Areas of enhancing soft tissue and bone are present in cases of maxillary periodontitis, alveolitis, and sinusitis (**Fig. 14**).

SUMMARY

CE-MRI is still in its infancy. The authors began using this technique as a way to improve understanding and push the limits of equine MRI. Contrast imaging provides a rich method of assessing the physiologic change that occurs in lesions detected with MRI. Further more rigorous clinical research from additional institutions will be necessary to evaluate and potentially establish this imaging technique as a valid component of equine MRI, particularly in musculoskeletal imaging. Following their initial clinical experiences, the authors strongly believe that CE-MRI is a valuable imaging tool in the assessment of the equine athlete.

REFERENCES

1. Ferrell EA, Gavin PR, Tucker RL, et al. Magnetic resonance for evaluation of neurologic disease in 12 horses. Vet Radiol Ultrasound 2002;43(6):510–6.
2. Tucker RL, Farrell E. Computed tomography and magnetic resonance imaging of the equine head. Vet Clin North Am Equine Pract 2001;17(1):131–44, vii.
3. Pekarkova M, Kircher PR, Konar M, et al. Magnetic resonance imaging anatomy of the normal equine larynx and pharynx. Vet Radiol Ultrasound 2009;50(4): 392–7.

4. Easley JT, Brokken MT, Zubrod CJ, et al. Magnetic resonance imaging findings in horses with septic arthritis. Vet Radiol Ultrasound 2011;52(4):402–8.
5. Judy CE. Contrast agents in equine MRI. In: Murray Rachel C, editor. Equine MRI. West Sussex (England): Wiley-Blackwell; 2011. p. 63–74.
6. Daniel AJ, Judy CE, Saveraid T. Magnetic resonance imaging of the metacarpo (tarso) phalangeal region in clinically lame horses responding to diagnostic analgesia of the palmar nerves at the base of the proximal sesamoid bones: five cases. Equine Vet Educ 2011.
7. Edelman Robert R, Hesselink John R, Zlatkin Michael B, Crues John V III, editors. Clinical magnetic resonance imaging. 3rd edition. Philadelphia: Elsevier Health Sciences; 2006.
8. Gavin PR, Bagley RS. Practical small animal MRI. Ames, Iowa: Wiley-Blackwell; 2009.
9. Judy C, Saveraid T, Rodgers E, et al. Characterization of foot lesions using contrast enhanced equine orthopedic magnetic resonance imaging. Proceedings of 2008 Veterinary Symposium. Germantown (MD): American College of Veterinary Surgeons. 2008.
10. Information on gadolinium-based contrast agents. Available at: http://www.fda.gov/drugs/drugsafety/postmarketdrugsafetyinformationforpatientsandproviders/ucm142882.htm. Accessed January 15, 2012.
11. Lin SP, Brown JJ. MR contrast agents: physical and pharmacologic basics. J Magn Reson Imaging 2007;25(5):884–99.
12. Weishaupt D, Köchli VD, Marinček B. How does MRI work?: an introduction to the physics and function of magnetic resonance imaging. 2nd edition. Berlin: Springer Verlag; 2006.
13. Kribben A, Witzke O, Hillen U, et al. Nephrogenic systemic fibrosis: pathogenesis, diagnosis, and therapy. J Am Coll Cardiol 2009;53(18):1621–8.
14. Hodgson RJ, Grainger AJ, O'Connor PJ, et al. Imaging of the Achilles tendon in spondyloarthritis: a comparison of ultrasound and conventional, short and ultrashort echo time MRI with and without intravenous contrast. Eur Radiol 2011;21(6):1144–52.
15. Denoix JM. The equine distal limb: atlas of clinical anatomy and comparative imaging. London: Thieme/Manson; 2000.
16. Murray RC. Equine MRI. West Sussex (England): Wiley-Blackwell; 2011.
17. Puchalski SM, Galuppo LD, Drew CP, et al. Use of contrast-enhanced computed tomography to assess angiogenesis in deep digital flexor tendinopathy in a horse. Vet Radiol Ultrasound 2009;50(3):292–7.
18. Vallance SA, Bell RJ, Spriet M, et al. Comparisons of computed tomography, contrast-enhanced computed tomography and standing low-field magnetic resonance imaging in horses with lameness localised to the foot. Part 2: Lesion identification. Equine Vet J 2012;44(2):149–56.
19. Smith RK. Pathophysiology of tendon injury. In: Ross MW, Dyson SJ, editors. Diagnosis and management of lameness in the horse. St Louis (MO): Saunders; 2003. p. 616–28.
20. Sharma P, Maffulli N. Biology of tendon injury: healing, modeling and remodeling. J Musculoskelet Neuronal Interact 2006;6(2):181–90.
21. Weinmann HJ, Brasch RC, Press WR, et al. Characteristics of gadolinium-DTPA complex: a potential NMR contrast agent. AJR Am J Roentgenol 1984;142(3):619–24.
22. Shalabi A, Kristoffersen-Wiberg M, Papadogiannakis N, et al. Dynamic contrast-enhanced MR imaging and histopathology in chronic Achilles tendinosis. A longitudinal MR study of 15 patients. Acta Radiol 2002;43(2):198–206.

23. Holowinski M, Judy C, Saveraid T, et al. Resolution of lesions on STIR images is associated with improved lameness status in horses. Vet Radiol Ultrasound 2010; 51(5):479–84.

24. Schramme M, Kerekes Z, Hunter S, et al. MR imaging features of surgically induced core lesions in the equine superficial digital flexor tendon. Vet Radiol Ultrasound 2010;51(3):280–7.

25. Maffulli N, Sharma P, Luscombe K. Achilles tendinopathy; aetiology and management. J R Soc Med 2004;97(10):472–6.

26. Spriet M, Mai W, McKnight A. Asymmetric signal intensity in normal collateral ligaments of the distal interphalangeal joint in horses with a low-field MRI system due to the magic angle effect. Vet Radiol Ultrasound 2007;48(2):95–100.

27. Spriet M, Zwingenberger A. Influence of the position of the foot on MRI signal in the deep digital flexor tendon and collateral ligaments of the distal interphalangeal joint in the standing horse. Equine Vet J 2009;41(5):498–503.

28. Werpy NM, Ho CP, Kawcak CE. Magic angle effect in normal collateral ligaments of the distal interphalangeal joint in horses imaged with a high-field magnetic resonance imaging system. Vet Radiol Ultrasound 2010;51(1):2–10.

29. Tehranzadeh J, Ashikyan O, Anavim A, et al. Enhanced MR imaging of tenosynovitis of hand and wrist in inflammatory arthritis. Skeletal Radiol 2006;35(11): 814–22.

30. MacMahon PJ, Eustace SJ, Kavanagh EC. Injectable corticosteroid and local anesthetic preparations: a review for radiologists. Radiology 2009;252(3):647–61.

31. Ostergaard M, Stoltenberg M, Henriksen O, et al. Quantitative assessment of synovial inflammation by dynamic gadolinium-enhanced magnetic resonance imaging. A study of the effect of intra-articular methylprednisolone on the rate of early synovial enhancement. Br J Rheumatol 1996;35(1):50–9.

32. Ostergaard M, Stoltenberg M, Lovgreen-Nielsen P, et al. Quantification of synovitis by MRI: correlation between dynamic and static gadolinium-enhanced magnetic resonance imaging and microscopic and macroscopic signs of synovial inflammation. Magn Reson Imaging 1998;16(7):743–54.

33. Ostergaard M, Klarlund M. Importance of timing of post-contrast MRI in rheumatoid arthritis: what happens during the first 60 minutes after IV gadolinium-DTPA? Ann Rheum Dis 2001;60(11):1050–4.

34. Lee JH, Dyke JP, Ballon D, et al. Assessment of bone perfusion with contrast-enhanced magnetic resonance imaging. Orthop Clin North Am 2009;40(2): 249–57.

35. Tehranzadeh J, Ashikyan O, Anavim A, et al. Detailed analysis of contrast-enhanced MRI of hands and wrists in patients with psoriatic arthritis. Skeletal Radiol 2008;37(5):433–42.

36. Fox MG, Stephens T, Jarjour WN, et al. Contrast-enhanced magnetic resonance imaging positively impacts the management of some patients with rheumatoid arthritis or suspected RA. J Clin Rheumatol 2012;18(1):15–22.

37. Ledermann HP, Morrison WB, Schweitzer ME. Pedal abscesses in patients suspected of having pedal osteomyelitis: analysis with MR imaging. Radiology 2002;224(3):649–55.

Biochemical Evaluation of Equine Articular Cartilage Through Imaging

Anthony Pease, DVM, MS, DACVR

KEYWORDS

• Equine • Cartilage • MRI • Imaging • Biochemical • Proteoglycan • Osteoarthritis

KEY POINTS

• Lameness causes a severe limitation to the quality and longevity of a horse's performance and show career.
• The metacarpophalangeal joint is a common site for cartilage damage in horses.
• Articular cartilage is the most difficult tissue to image in the diarthrodial joint.
• Magnetic resonance imaging is becoming the gold standard for evaluation of the soft tissues of the equine limb.

Lameness causes a severe limitation to the quality and longevity of a horse's performance and show career. The American Association of Equine Practitioners conducted a survey in 2009 of more than 6000 equine practitioners to identify the top research priorities for the equine industry. The musculoskeletal system was listed as having the highest research priority, with exercise-related diseases considered the most important.[1] Because of this need, numerous research studies associated with magnetic resonance imaging (MRI) of articular cartilage have been conducted. Recently, several studies using standard imaging techniques to evaluate articular cartilage in high- and low-strength magnets have been published for animals.[2] In addition, the use of molecular MRI in horses and animals is just beginning to be performed, despite use in human medicine for more than 10 years.[3–6]

The metacarpophalangeal joint is a common site for cartilage damage in horses. The metacarpophalangeal joint in the young equine athlete is a high-motion joint that experiences considerable loads during exercise, which can lead to a condition known as overload arthrosis.[7] Because of a predisposition for joint disease at this location, numerous studies have been performed to try to identify early signs of this

No financial support was received for this data.
Author has nothing to disclose.
Veterinary Diagnostic Imaging, College of Veterinary Medicine, Michigan State University, East Lansing, MI 48824, USA
E-mail address: peasean@cvm.msu.edu

disease.[2, 7–10] Conventional wisdom holds that early lesions in the articular cartilage and subchondral bone are generally asymptomatic and lameness is not observed until more advanced and potentially irreparable changes in the cartilage and subchondral bone have occurred. Indeed, catastrophic failure has been seen in horses with few if any significant pre-existing signs using standard imaging. After early cartilage damage, the loss of proteoglycans, and disruption of the collagen network, the capacity of cartilage to resist load is reduced and leads to additional fibrillation, even during physiologic loading.[11] Detection of lesions before more advanced cartilage degeneration is essential if prevention or repair of damaged cartilage is to occur. Other joints also get osteoarthritis; however, the metacarpophalangeal joint is well suited for MRI and the current standard of radiographic or even MRI looking for osteophytosis or irregularities in the articular cartilage margin would already indicate irreparable damage to the joint.[2]

Articular cartilage is the most difficult tissue to image in the diarthrodial joint. Although ligaments surrounding the joint and the synovial lining can be characterized ultrasonographically, the evaluation of the articular cartilage is limited to the non–weight-bearing surfaces and artifacts because of the curvature of the joint surface. In the metacarpophalangeal joint, the proximal sesamoid bones also provide a barrier to imaging the articular surface of the palmar aspect of the distal condyles. In the proximal and distal interphalangeal joints, very limited areas of joint surfaces can be seen because of the close apposition of bone, similar to the carpus and tarsus. Stifle and shoulder joints have limited information available because of the lack of clinical computed tomographic and MRI units that can perform this procedure. Despite this limitation, some studies have compared positive contrast medium arthrography of the stifle joint with gross pathology and the stifle anatomy on MRI; however, most of these studies are performed on cadaver limbs. Computed tomography (CT) scans and radiographs cannot differentiate soft tissue and fluid, although using arthrography, a limited assessment of the margin of the articular surface is possible. Recently, CT with contrast medium enhancement was used to detect degenerative cartilage in human cadaver specimens, but no tests using CT in live humans or in veterinary medicine to assess the molecular properties of articular cartilage have been performed and the usefulness of contrast-enhanced CT is unknown.[12] The most definitive diagnostic and therapeutic method to evaluate the cartilage surface in a joint is with arthroscopy. Although atraumatic compared with arthrotomy, convalescent time is required before returning to training. In addition, arthroscopic access to some clinically relevant areas is limited and the assessment mainly looks at the surface contour and underestimates the severity of disease with mild cartilage damage, whereas overestimating the extent of disease with more established lesions.[13]

MRI is becoming the gold standard for evaluation of the soft tissues of the equine limb.[2] The superior resolution of pathologic changes to tendons, bones, and articular cartilage provides a noninvasive window into the pathologic anatomy of an articular joint.[2, 7–10] However, standard MRI sequences only provide anatomic information on the articular cartilage surface.[2,10] In humans, it is recommended to acquire images using magnets with a field strength of 1.5 T or greater and to use a slice thickness of 1 to 2 mm to maximize the resolution of articular cartilage.[14] In horses, low-field standing magnets have typically been used to identify cartilage defects, but only the most severe lesions are evident and many less severe lesions are not detected.[15–17] The low-field-strength systems lack the resolution to identify subtle defects in articular cartilage and the image acquisition time is limited when relevant slice thicknesses are desired, even if general anesthesia is used. One concern has been that using high-field-strength systems, general anesthesia is needed. However, recovery from anesthesia in these patients poses a minimal risk and MRI procedures in horses are being performed as part of a routine standard of care for difficult lameness evaluations. In addition, with current high-field-strength systems and imaging sequences, the image acquisition and interpretation focuses on the identification of cartilage defects and fibrillation, an irreversible change that can be career limiting for a high-level equine athlete at the time of detection. Because of the minimal thickness of the articular cartilage in the equine joint compared with humans, the ability to see surface lesions is not possible unless a large amount of synovial fluid is present to provide an interface between the two opposing joint surfaces. In addition, linear defects and small defects that are less than the slice thickness of the MRI cannot be seen. This limitation is based on the idea that larger slice thicknesses (>2 mm) are needed to image the equine limb to minimize time while maintaining adequate signal to make a diagnostic image. In standing and recumbent MRI units, the trade-off is always present between the time needed to get the sequence and the time the patient needs to stand still or can be under general anesthesia without causing complications, such as motion artifact or muscle damage.[2] Despite these limitations, high-field-strength MRI (≥1 T) is still considered the modality of choice to evaluate the articular cartilage of horses, mainly because a more suitable method to assess the health of articular cartilage does not yet exist and the ability for high-resolution, thin slice acquisition in a short time frame is only available in high-field-strength systems.

Loss of proteoglycans within the cartilage matrix is considered to be among the first pathophysiologic events in osteoarthritis. This proteoglycan loss is something that specialized MRI sequences should be able to identify noninvasively.[18] In humans, specialized molecular imaging sequences, such as delayed gadolinium-enhanced MRI of cartilage (dGEMRIC), have detected early changes in the proteoglycan content of articular cartilage in patients with osteoarthritis,[14] and sequential imaging of the articular cartilage using dGEMRIC has been used to monitor improvements in the biochemical status of human cartilage in trauma or joint surgery patients undergoing physiotherapy.[19] The premise that changes in cartilage proteoglycan content might be detected with an accuracy approaching that of histopathologic evaluation holds considerable promise.[18]

APPEARANCE OF JOINTS USING DIFFERENT SEQUENCES

MRI focuses on the imaging of hydrogen atoms, which are the most abundant in the body, to generate an image. Using this atom, all image sequences are based on the appearance of water. T1 or tissue 1 characteristics compared with T2 or tissue 2 characteristics are the basic weightings on which all image sequences in MRI are based. The physics behind these sequences is beyond the scope of this artical, but basically, T1 characteristics highlight soft tissues and do not show fluid and are generally considered sequences for anatomy, whereas T2 weighting is centered on fluid and is primarily used to image pathology. Manipulation of the T1 and T2 weightings is performed to highlight articular cartilage, which is primarily made of water, compared with the adjacent synovial fluid and the subchondral bone to evaluate for pathology.

Unfortunately, no one sequence is considered superior to all others when it comes to imaging the equine joint. The various image sequences have a characteristic appearance (**Fig. 1**). Therefore, multiple images sequences and image planes are needed for a complete examination. Parameters, such as slice thickness, magnet strength, and patient size, all have bearing on the image quality that is produced. However, some basic trends do apply. On T1-weighted images, gradient echo sequences, primarily those that are fat suppressed, have the ability to acquire images

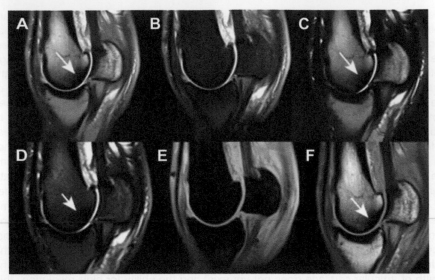

Fig. 1. Sagittal images of the metacarpophalangeal joint using multiple image sequences. (*A*) Proton density. (*B*) Proton density with fat saturation. (*C*) Short tau inversion recovery. (*D*) T2-weighted image. (*E*) T1 VIBE. (*F*) T1-weighted image. These images show the range of sequences available. Note that on images *A, C, D,* and *F* subchondral sclerosis is identified (*arrow*).

rapidly and can have thin slice thickness. In humans, this sequence was shown to have 94% sensitivity for detecting cartilage defects compared with arthroscopy, but T2-weighted sequences and standard T1-weighted sequences had 93% sensitivity.[20] In veterinary medicine, the larger the lesion, the more likely it is detected. The size and shape of articular cartilage and subchondral bone defects were most accurately demonstrated on low-field T2-weighted fast spin echo images and on high-field proton-density and T2-weighted fast spin echo images.[2] Certain sequences, such as the T2* gradient echo sequence, on low-field-strength systems did not demonstrate any lesions.[2] Using a standard T1 fat-suppressed gradient echo sequence does provide good contrast between the mild signal from the fat of subchondral bone and the articular cartilage. However, the articular cartilage surface is difficult to assess because of the presence and summation with the surrounding synovial fluid.

Newer T1 gradient echo sequences called ultrafast gradient echo (VIBE or Turbo-FLASH, Siemens, Melvern; THRIVE, Phillips, Andover; Fast SPGR, General Electric, Wauwatosa), provide much better evaluation of the articular. Unlike standard gradient echo sequences, the ultrafast gradient echo provides images where the bone is severely dark because of very low signal, but the difference between the articular cartilage surface and the synovial fluid is quite separate allowing for excellent articular cartilage conspicuity.

Proton-density images provide a bridge maximizing T1 characteristics while providing a small amount of T2 data. This is done by having a slightly longer TE than a T1-weighted image (~30–35 milliseconds), while having a much long TR than a T1-weighted sequence (>1500 milliseconds). This allows for maximum T2 relaxation to optimize T1 and T2 weighting. The proton-density sequence was found to be best for evaluating articular cartilage in one study of horses comparing articular cartilage defects using various sequences and magnets because it provided the best overall assessment of the subchondral bone, articular cartilage, and synovial fluid.[9]

However, the low-signal-intensity articular cartilage on T2-weighted fast spin echo sequences summates with the subchondral bone creating a thicker region of low signal intensity at the articular surface. This appearance can be helpful in identifying small or shallow articular cartilage defects that contrast with adjacent high-signal-intensity synovial fluid.

Short tau inversion recovery sequences also provide good anatomic information, but because of a relative lack of signal, these sequences are much preferred to identify bone edema. Articular cartilage can often be more easily identified when there is overlying synovial fluid. The synovial fluid fills articular cartilage defects or region of thinning increasing the visibility of these lesions. When the articular surfaces contact the conspicuity of the cartilage margins, any associated abnormalities are reduced.

Contrast Media for MRI are Made of Negatively Charged Ions

Gadobenate dimeglumine (Gd-BOPTA, 529 mg/mL; MultiHance, Bracco Diagnostic, Princeton, NJ) or gadopentate dimeglumine (Gd-DTPA; Magnevist, Wayne, NJ) are negative charged, which is important because proteoglycans within articular cartilage are also negatively charged.[21,22] As a result, contrast medium are excluded from healthy cartilage matrix. When proteoglycans are lost from the extracellular matrix, the negative charge of the articular cartilage decreases, allowing proportional uptake of contrast medium. Although this enhancement is not evident on conventional monitors, it can be quantified using specialized analysis software, such as MatLab (Natick, Massachusetts) or other such statistical programs. Two methods are used. One is based on multiple inversion time T1 measurements creating a T1 map (**Fig. 2**), whereas it has also been suggested that running a T2-weighted image before and after administration of contrast medium could also be used to deduce contrast medium concentrations within the articular cartilage using one sequence instead of specialized software.[22] The charge of the contrast medium only controls the amount of contrast medium that diffuses into the articular cartilage, but not the spatial diffusion of the contrast medium within the cartilage, which remains inhomogenous across the thickness of the articular cartilage.[22]

The Basis of dGEMRIC Imaging is the Presence of Equilibrium

Because of the negative charge of the articular cartilage and the negative charge of the MR contrast medium, the normal repulsion between these two structures limits the changes seen within the cartilage matrix. Ex vivo studies using dGEMRIC indicate that equilibrium between the cartilage and the contrast medium is established and, as a result, provides uniform reproducible results.[12] When cartilage is normal (**Fig. 3**), then the contrast medium has minimal ability to penetrate to the level of the subchondral bone. As the cartilage losses the proteoglycan matrix (**Fig. 4**), the contrast medium is no longer repelled and can be detected using specialized software (see **Fig. 2**). In a living animal, the contrast medium is constantly circulated so that the time required to establish this equilibrium is variable. Factors that influence the rate of equilibration include the vascular distribution of the contrast medium and the thickness of the articular cartilage. As a result, in humans, a typical protocol for dGEMRIC of the knee and peripheral structures involves a double dose of contrast medium followed by 15 minutes of light exercise and then scanning at 2 to 3 hours after contrast medium administration.[5] In the horse, a double dose of contrast medium (generally 40 mL or 0.2 mmol/kg) has been administered intravenously and then passive motion of the joint was performed for 30 minutes. Alternatively, administering the contrast medium before induction and exercising the horse can be performed to allow equilibrium of contrast medium into the synovial fluid and penetration into the joint to occur.

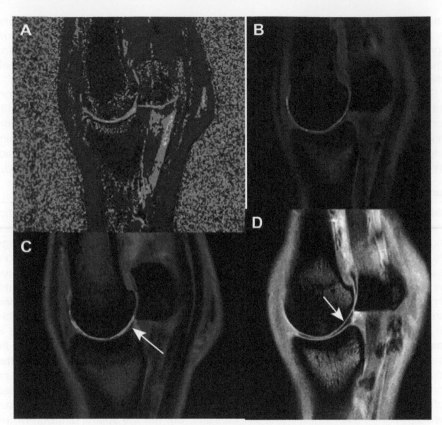

Fig. 2. (*A*) Color map generated using the dGEMRIC protocol. This map shows a diversity of colors based on the signal intensity obtained during the image acquisition. (*B*) Fused image of a normal metacarpophalangeal joint with a contoured cartilage dGEMRIC map over an anatomic scan. Note the uniform blue color throughout the palmar region of the cartilage map. (*C*) Fused image of a cartilage dGEMRIC map over an anatomic scan in a horse with clinical lameness localized to the metacarpophalangeal joint. Notice the red region at the palmar aspect of the cartilage map indicating increased contrast medium uptake caused by loss of proteoglycans. (*D*) Standard MRI T1-weighted image of the same specimen as **Fig. 1C** showing subchondral sclerosis (decreased signal) in the mid-palmar aspect of the condyle. Notice that the articular cartilage (*arrow*) has a uniform appearance. This scan fails to reveal articular cartilage damage, but does show signs secondary to osteoarthritis.

T2 Mapping, T1ρ, dGEMRIC MRI Sequences, and CT

dGEMRIC is not the only method to evaluate the articular cartilage. Specialized T2 cartilage maps have been correlated with tissue hydration and have been shown to inversely correlate with cartilage volume and thickness. Generally, early osteoarthritic changes in T2 are related to change in the collagen content of articular cartilage, but do not correlate with proteoglycan loss according to the literature.[12] T1ρ is a method to evaluate the spin-lattice energy exchange between water and large molecules that comprise the extracellular matrix of articular cartilage.[12] By disrupting this matrix through loss of the proteoglycan content, water molecules have increased motion that causes increases to T1ρ measurements.[23] T1 dGEMRIC and contrast medium-enhanced CT can also be used to indirectly evaluate the proteoglycan content.

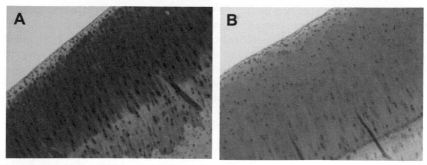

Fig. 3. Digital images of the articular cartilage of an equine third metacarpal bone in the mid-palmar region stained with alcian blue (*A*) and safranin O (*B*). Note the uniform intensity of the staining in both slides (original magnification ×5).

Both methods use a negatively charged contrast medium agent and with CT, the method is rapid and can be directly measured using Hounsfield units.[24] Because of the limited volume of contrast medium within the joint, higher contrast medium doses are generally used with CT and MRI. Contrast medium–enhanced CT is proposed to have the potential advantage of being a direct measure of contrast medium based on the sensing electron density rather than MRI, which indirectly measures the relaxation time of tissue that is being affected by the contrast-medium.[12] Also, because relaxation times are affected by inhomogeneities in the magnetic field, absolute quantification is difficult, especially among patients.[12] Because most damage to equine cartilage is focal, especially in the metacarpophalangeal joint, the remaining cartilage or contralateral aspect of the condyle potentially serves as an internal control. Comparison of all these techniques using cartilage explants found that precontrast medium T1ρ and dGEMRIC had a low correlation, meaning that there may be more to early osteoarthritis loss than proteoglycan degradation. The precontrast medium T2 values did not correlate with any other imaging measure, meaning that hydration may provide complimentary information beyond what is gained from dGEMRIC. The most interesting finding in this study was the moderate correlation between contrast medium–enhanced CT and dGEMRIC. This decreased correlation is believed to show the other causes of inhomogeneity found with MRI compared with the absolute

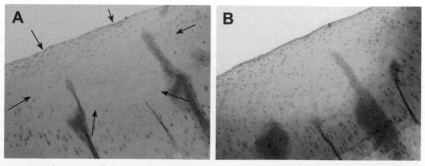

Fig. 4. Digital images of the articular cartilage in the mid-palmar region of the same equine as **Fig. 3**, but opposite third metacarpal bone. There is a marked loss of proteoglycan content evident with alcian blue (*A; arrows*) and safranin O (*B*); however, the loss is more readily identified with safranin O staining (original magnification ×5).

Hounsfield attenuation obtained by CT.[12] Practical considerations of anesthesia time make T2 precontrast medium imaging more difficult; however, in ponies, precontrast medium images were obtained, then contrast medium administered after 30 minutes range of motion exercise before postcontrast medium imaging.[2] However, using postcontrast medium dGEMRIC alone may lead to an overestimation of the proteoglycan concentration, especially in repair tissue.[25] Also, T2 mapping is thought to have limited potential to assess specific biochemical markers in native cartilage and repair tissue.[3]

LIMITATIONS OF MRI AND CARTILAGE

The largest limitation of imaging (MRI or CT) to evaluate the articular cartilage is slice thickness. The lower the field strength of the magnet, the thicker the slice acquired and the larger the defects need to be before they can be resolved. CT, especially multislice machines, has the benefit of smaller slice thickness and rapid speed, but without contrast medium within the joint, soft tissue and fluid appear the same and articular cartilage evaluation is limited. Despite this limitation, identifying subchondral sclerosis is easily seen and the evaluation of pathology in the equine joint using CT or MRI is considered far superior compared with digital images because of the lack of superimposition and increased contrast resolution of cross-sectional modalities.[26] Ultrasound evaluation of articular cartilage is very angle dependent and because it cannot assess the weight-bearing surfaces and the limited ability to image around sesamoid bones where ebernation occurs, the use of ultrasound in horses is mainly limited to evaluation for joint effusion, ligament and meniscal tears, and synovial proliferation. MRI is very diverse with artifacts occurring not just because of motion on a low-field-strength system, but also the limitation that low-field magnets require an increased amount of time to obtain image resolution seen on the higher-strength systems. Motion artifact, despite correction software, causes blurring of images, making the ability to evaluate subtle, 1-mm defects in articular cartilage nearly impossible. MRI is always a balance between sequence selection, imaging plane, and slice thickness to maximize image resolution and minimize scanning time. A set protocol for imaging of the equine skeleton that provides the maximum chance for lesion identification is greatly needed, but difficult to agree on.

SUMMARY

Ultimately, the use of molecular imaging of cartilage is the next vital step in understanding, treating, and training the equine athlete. Because of the logistics of precontrast and postcontrast medium imaging, the clinical usefulness of the examination has come into question.[4] That said, with the large number of horses undergoing high-field MRI, the use of contrast medium administration and T1 mapping or T2 imaging precontrast and postcontrast medium administration may add a very limited amount of extra time to the scan and has the potential to provide more detailed information about the chemical composition of the articular cartilage that is not seen with routine imaging.

REFERENCES

1. AAEP, Foundation. Membership Equine Research Study. 2009. Available at: http://www.aaep.org/images/files/Research%20Study%20-%20Final%20-%2010%2007%2009.pdf.
2. Menendez MI, Clark DJ, Carlton M, et al. Direct delayed human adenoviral BMP-2 or BMP-6 gene therapy for bone and cartilage regeneration in a pony osteochondral model. Osteoarthritis Cartilage 2011;19(8):1066–75.

3. Watanabe A, Boesch C, Anderson SE, et al. Ability of dGEMRIC and T2 mapping to evaluate cartilage repair after microfracture: a goat study. Osteoarthritis Cartilage 2009;17(10):1341–9.
4. Burstein D, Velyvis J, Scott KT, et al. Protocol issues for delayed Gd(DTPA)(2-)-enhanced MRI (dGEMRIC) for clinical evaluation of articular cartilage. Magn Reson Med 2001;45(1):36–41.
5. Trattnig S, Winalski CS, Marlovits S, et al. Magnetic resonance imaging of cartilage repair: a review. Cartilage 2011;2(1):5–26.
6. Norrdin RW, Bay BK, Drews MJ, et al. Overload arthrosis: strain patterns in the equine metacarpal condyle. J Musculoskelet Neuronal Interact 2001;1(4):357–62.
7. Brama PA, Tekoppele JM, Bank RA, et al. Topographical mapping of biochemical properties of articular cartilage in the equine fetlock joint. Equine Vet J 2000;32(1):19–26.
8. Dyson S, Murray R, Schramme M, et al. Magnetic resonance imaging of the equine foot: 15 horses. Equine Vet J 2003;35(1):18–26.
9. Werpy N, Ho C, Pease A, et al. Detection of osteochondral defects in the fetlock joint using low and high field strength MR imaging and the effect of sequence selection. Vet Radiol Ultrasound 2011;52(2):154–60.
10. Olive J, D'Anjou MA, Alexander K, et al. Comparison of magnetic resonance imaging, computed tomography, and radiography for assessment of noncartilaginous changes in equine metacarpophalangeal osteoarthritis. Vet Radiol Ultrasound 2010;51(3):267–79.
11. Bekkers JE, Creemers LB, Dhert WJ, et al. Diagnostic modalities for diseased articular cartilage—from defect to degeneration: a review. Cartilage 2010;1(3):157–64.
12. Taylor C, Carballido-Gamio J, Majumdar S, et al. Comparison of quantitative imaging of cartilage for osteoarthritis: T2, T1ρ, dGEMRIC and contrast-enhanced computed tomography. Magn Reson Imaging 2009;27:779–84.
13. Brommer H, Rijkenhuizen AB, Brama PA, et al. Accuracy of diagnostic arthroscopy for the assessment of cartilage damage in the equine metacarpophalangeal joint. Equine Vet J 2004;36(4):331–5.
14. Jazrawi LM, Alaia MJ, Chang G, et al. Advances in magnetic resonance imaging of articular cartilage. J Am Acad Orthop Surg 2011;19(7):420–9.
15. Murray RC, Mair TS, Sherlock CE, et al. Comparison of high-field and low-field magnetic resonance images of cadaver limbs of horses. Vet Rec 2009;165(10):281–8.
16. Olive J. Distal interphalangeal articular cartilage assessment using low-field magnetic resonance imaging. Vet Radiol Ultrasound 2010;51(3):259–66.
17. Sherlock CE, Mair TS, Ter Braake F. Osseous lesions in the metacarpo(tarso)phalangeal joint diagnosed using low-field magnetic resonance imaging in standing horses. Vet Radiol Ultrasound 2009;50(1):13–20.
18. Deborah B, Martha G, Tim M, et al. Measures of molecular composition and structure in osteoarthritis. Radiol Clin North Am 2009;47(4):675–86.
19. Burstein D. Tracking longitudinal changes in knee degeneration and repair. J Bone Joint Surg Am 2009;91(Suppl 1):51–3.
20. Disler DG, McCauley TR, Wirth CR, et al. Detection of knee hyaline cartilage defects using fat-suppressed three-dimensional spoiled gradient-echo MR imaging: comparison with standard MR imaging and correlation with arthroscopy. AJR Am J Roentgenol 1995;165(2):377–82.
21. Maroudas A. Distribution and diffusion of solutes in articular cartilage. Biophys J 1970;10(5):365–79.

22. Wiener E, Woertler K, Weirich G, et al. Contrast enhanced cartilage imaging: comparison of ionic and non-ionic contrast agents. Eur J Radiol 2007;63(1): 110–9.
23. Regatte RR, Akella SV, Borthakur A, et al. In vivo proton MR three-dimensional T1rho mapping of human articular cartilage: initial experience. Radiology 2003; 229(1):269–74.
24. Cockman MD, Blanton CA, Chmielewski PA, et al. Quantitative imaging of proteo-glycan in cartilage using a gadolinium probe and microCT. Osteoarthritis Carti-lage 2006;14(3):210–4.
25. Watanabe A, Wada Y, Obata T, et al. Delayed gadolinium-enhanced MR to deter-mine glycosaminoglycan concentration in reparative cartilage after autologous chondrocyte implantation: preliminary results. Radiology 2006;239(1):201–8.
26. O'Brien T, Baker TA, Brounts SH, et al. Detection of articular pathology of the distal aspect of the third metacarpal bone in thoroughbred racehorses: compar-ison of radiography, computed tomography and magnetic resonance imaging. Vet Surg 2011;40(8):942–51.

The Role of MRI in Selected Equine Case Management

Myra F. Barrett, DVM, MS[a],*, David D. Frisbie, DVM, PhD[b]

KEYWORDS

- MRI - Equine - Case management - Orthopedics

KEY POINTS

- MRI allows for the diagnosis of bone, joints, and soft tissue pathologic change.
- Using MRI as a diagnostic modality can aid in the development of case-specific treatment protocols.
- Treatment protocols can include surgical intervention, intralesional and perilesional therapy, use of various biologic agents, and other medical management.
- An individualized and accurately formed treatment plan provides the best opportunity for a successful outcome.

INTRODUCTION

The value of MRI for diagnosis of equine musculoskeletal injuries has been established in the literature and clinical practice, and continues to be explored. MRI can be used to identify injuries that are not detected using other imaging modalities or to provide more complete characterization of known pathologic change.

MRI is particularly useful for examining soft tissue structures that cannot be completely assessed with ultrasound, such as the collateral ligaments of the distal interphalangeal (DIP) joint, and is the superior modality for assessing articular cartilage and many forms of bone pathology. The detail that MRI can provide regarding extent, type, severity and, in some cases, chronicity of injury is useful from a diagnostic standpoint as well as for guiding therapeutic intervention. This article aims to explore the ways in which MRI aids in the case management of various types of musculoskeletal injuries.

David Frisbie is a consultant for Arthrex and a partner in Advanced Regenerative Technologies, a bone marrow-derived stem cell company.
[a] Department of Environmental and Radiological Health Sciences, Veterinary Teaching Hospital, Colorado State University, 300 West Drake, Fort Collins, CO 80523, USA;
[b] Department of Clinical Sciences, Gail Holmes Equine Orthopaedic Research Center, Colorado State University, 300 West Drake, Fort Collins, CO 80523, USA
* Corresponding author.
E-mail address: myra@colostate.edu

JOINT DISEASE

High field strength (≥1 T) MRI is the superior imaging modality for examining articular cartilage and is frequently used to assess structural changes in cartilage. Because MRI is a noninvasive diagnostic technique, it is frequently used as a presurgical diagnostic modality in humans. Likewise, in equine patients, although general anesthesia is often still required, MRI is an excellent noninvasive method to assess joints. MRI allows for evaluation of cartilage, subchondral bone, and both intra-articular and extra-articular soft tissues, including interarticular ligaments such as the intercarpal ligaments, joint capsule, and collateral ligaments. Additionally, although some parts of joints are not accessible arthroscopically or ultrasonographically, MRI provides a complete image of the joint.

Medical Management

MRI may reveal articular cartilage damage in a location that cannot be accessed via arthroscopy, and thereby circumvent an unnecessary surgery. In such cases, medical management can be directed by the MRI findings. Intra-articular biologic therapy such as, autologous conditioned serum (ACS; IRAP II) and bone marrow-derived stems cells (BMSC) is often indicated in such cases, after routine therapeutic measures have been taken (**Fig. 1**).

In addition to the evaluation of cartilage, MRI promotes detection of subchondral bone sclerosis, cystic lesions, osseous hyperintensity secondary to edema, inflammatory infiltrate, hemorrhage, or necrosis. Medical treatment of these conditions includes regional intravenous (IV) perfusion with stem cell therapy or in some cases tiludronate (Tildren).

Because of historic difficulties in imaging the soft tissue in and around the joint, it has often been overlooked as a cause of lameness. For example, a relatively common

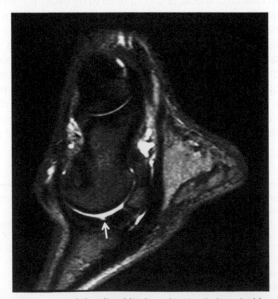

Fig. 1. Parasagittal STIR image of the distal limb. A focal subchondral bone defect is present in mid-palmar P3. This area cannot be visualized arthroscopically. The patient was treated with intra-articular BMSC therapy with a positive response to therapy.

source of lameness is desmopathy of the collateral ligaments of the DIP joint.[1,2] Only the proximal portion of the collateral ligaments of the DIP can be assessed ultrasonographically, and radiographic evaluation of the collateral fossae on the third phalanx can be challenging. Therefore, MRI is a particularly valuable tool for assessment of the ligaments themselves and the osseous origin and insertion.

Treatment of desmopathy and enthesopathy of the collateral ligaments will vary depending the type, location, and extent of the lesion. In the authors' experience, milder lesions can benefit from focused extracorporeal shockwave therapy. Although this is an attractive treatment modality because of its noninvasive nature, many cases can benefit from aggressive intralesional and/or perilesional therapies such as BMSC or platelet-rich plasma (PRP). Lesions of the collateral ligaments of the DIP that are more proximally located can be treated with ultrasound guidance. In general, intralesional injections are reserved for discrete tears or core lesions, whereas periligamentous treatment is used in cases of diffuse damage, enlargement, or degenerative changes. In the authors' opinion, repeat intralesional injections in a healing tear are contraindicated because of the risk of damaging the repairing tissue scaffold.

Intralesional therapy is also indicated for tearing or desmopathy of the portion of the collateral ligaments within the hoof capsule, as well as for resorptive or cystic lesions of the collateral ligament fossae on the distal phalanx. Due to the location within the hoof capsule, this cannot be performed with ultrasound guidance. In these cases, radiographic-guided needle placement is recommended. The findings of the MRI will help direct the needle to the placement in a medial to lateral direction as well as a cranial to caudal direction (**Fig. 2**).[3]

Surgical Management

Arthroscopy
Using traditional diagnostics, cartilage damage is often not diagnosed until secondary signs, such as osteophytes or other evidence of joint disease, are detected on radiographic or ultrasonographic examination. Early detection of cartilage damage with MRI and subsequent therapeutic intervention, such as subchondral bone microfracture (aka micropicking), can help prevent progression of joint disease. More specifically, untreated articular cartilage lesions can often continue to shed debris in to the joint space. This debris is thought to be integral in perpetuating the proinflammatory cascade by the synovium.[4] Thus, early debridement of cartilage lesions may aid in returning the joint environment to a more normal state, slowing down the progression of osteoarthritis.

Arthrodesis
Many joints can be diagnosed as end-stage joint disease based on radiographic findings, which can include joint space narrowing, subchondral bone lysis and sclerosis, and marked periarticular osteophytosis and remodeling. In such cases, the need for therapeutic intervention involving arthrodesis is often clear. However, determining the appropriate timing of tarsal arthrodesis can more challenging based on radiographic examination. In part, this is because there is a lack of consistent correlation between radiographic abnormalities and clinical disease. It is also confounded by the lack of definitive diagnostic anesthesia in this region; distal tarsal disease and proximal suspensory ligament disease often result in a similar blocking pattern. Therefore, ruling out suspensory ligament disease is important and the proximal suspensory ligament should be included in the MRI examination of the distal tarsus. In the authors' experience, the severity of subchondral bone disease is often the most sensitive indication of the degree of tarsal disease as it relates to clinical signs. Further, pathologic

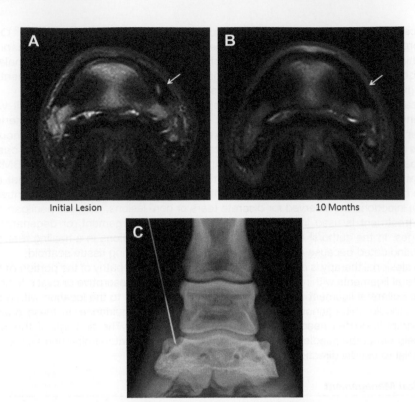

Fig. 2. (*A*) Initial transverse proton density MR image demonstrating an area of marked hyperintensity and enlargement of the distal aspect of the lateral collateral ligament of the distal interphalangeal joint (*white arrow*), indicating severe fiber disruption. (*B*) 10-month follow-up transverse proton density MRI at the same level as (*A*). The lateral collateral ligament show marked healing (*white arrow*), as seen by the significant decrease in size and signal intensity. (*C*) Horizontal dorsopalmar radiograph demonstrating the approach for radiographic-guided intralesional therapy at the insertion of the collateral ligament of the distal interphalangeal joint. ([*C*] *Data from* Werpy N, Farrington L, Frisbie D. How to perform radiographic-guided needle placement into the collateral ligaments of the distal interphalangel joint. vol. 57. San Antonio (TX): American Association of Equine Practitioners; 2011. p. 451–5; and *Reprinted from* American Association of Equine Practitioners; with permission.)

change of the subchondral and trabecular bone is often underestimated based on radiographic examination. Specifically, subchondral bone defects, cartilage loss, cystic lesions, sclerosis, bone edema, and osteonecrosis are all possible findings that can be undetected or underestimated with radiographs. Understanding the extent of subchondral disease based on MRI examination can help more readily identify horses that are unlikely to be manageable with intra-articular medication and may benefit from arthrodesis of the distal tarsal joints.

TENOSYNOVITIS

The underlying source of pain in lameness that has been localized to the digital sheath can be frustrating to determine. MRI can detect subtle tears, particularly in areas that